The Blueprint Method

A New Miasmatic Map &
Method of Prescribing for Homeopaths
That Transcends the Influences of the
Modern World

Danica Apolline-Matić

First Published in Great Britain in 2024 by
Danica Apolline-Matić

978-0-9575721-7-1

Dedicated to Dr Samuel Hahnemann, the Ultimate Pioneer, who taught us to keep growing and evolving and finding new ways to address the challenges we face.

Contents

Acknowledgements

I am hugely grateful to the remarkable homeopaths that inspire me every day. Especially my dear friends and colleagues in the Golden Spiral Provings Collective: Eugénie Krüger, Sarah Valentini, Reeta Pohjonen, Andrea Szekely, Wanda Whiting, Daniel Burge, Gosia Charysz, Hilery Hampel, Joy Ellis, Dr Paul Theriault, Rebecca Dove-Thomas, Rasunah Sellars, Sally Moore, Siobhan Purcell. Also my brilliant Golden Spiral School of Homeopathy sisters Lisa Strbac and Ramona Popescu.

An extra special thank you to Nick Biggins, Janey Lavelle and Ian Watson for taking the time to go through earlier drafts and giving fantastic feedback.

A huge thank you to the patients I see and have seen, who also inspire me greatly. I am in constant awe of the power of the human spirit, and the strength of the vital force, through what they teach me, and show me.

My heartfelt gratitude to teachers, and colleagues, whose lessons and wisdoms I carry in my heart.

My dear friends, who continue to encourage me always. You know who you are. I love you.

My beautiful son, who proved to me that homeopathy wasn't, as I had believed, a placebo.

And a massive thank you to Val Lawrence, one of the kindest, humblest, most brilliant teachers, who made my journey into homeopathy possible.

"Your soul is the whole world"

- Hermann Hesse

Introduction

We live in unprecedented times with an invitation to grow beyond the more challenging influences created by humankind.

There is a calling to return to living in a way that we all once knew - in harmony with the whole of our being, with the plants, trees, animals and planet; a return to remembering ourselves as whole, and connected to every aspect of ourselves and the world around us.

We are being invited to remember who and what we really are: energetic beings.

The Blueprint Method is an invitation to work with remedies that connect us at a level needed for these times of transformation – to our own energetic matrix ourselves and through that to each other, and to our beautiful world.

The Blueprint Method invites us to consciously work with our energetic matrix, using remedies that enable us to transcend physical, emotional, mental & spiritual traumas and that bring a return to wholeness in the very fabric of our being - our energetic blueprint.

This is the next level of working with sarcodes; working with the greatest organ we have. Our energy field.

The Journey to the Blueprint

In December 2020, the Golden Spiral Provings Collective carried out a proving of the Epstein-Barr Virus (EBV), during which it became clear that EBV is a miasm. This led to a revisiting of miasms more broadly in the context of our modern world.

From this I proposed the first draft of a new Miasmatic Map, that has since evolved into what I present here. It reflects the world we currently find ourselves in, and brings with it a new understanding of how to build on remarkable existing methods to treat the pathologies we find, and support a return to wholeness in health.

In order to explain how this new method has evolved, it feels important to revisit the fundamental tenets of miasms and sarcodes - and the very philosophy that influenced Dr Hahnemann in his quest to find a safer, kinder form of medicine that works. We begin our journey with another look at miasms, and how they have been rapidly expanding in our world.

Miasms

When I came across miasms as a student, I believed them to be a concept unique to homeopathy; another wonderful word that came from days of old that it was important to learn. Even though I was taught that there was a historical meaning to the term miasm that comes from the Greek language, meaning taint or pollution, I had no idea that Dr Samuel Hahnemann was using a term that was commonly understood in his time – a phrase that can be linked to being an expression of Antoine Beauchamp's Terrain Theory.

The original miasms, as written about by Dr Hahnemann, all come from disease processes that are known as the "taints" or "pollutants".

As Ian Watson describes in his wonderful book The Homeopathic Miasms: A Modern View, Dr Hahnemann had already begun prescribing using an "anti-miasmatic" approach, alongside another remedy to treat the symptoms that were presenting themselves, believing it to be a challenge for the vital force to overcome the "negative morbific influence" of the miasms. Ian discusses his perceptive realisation that "miasmatic theory in its original form is really a branch of allopathic thinking hidden within homeopathy". In trying to get rid of the miasm, we are, Ian suggests, aligning more with a Germ Theory perspective.

Ian also introduces a insightful and holistic way of thinking about miasms, suggesting that it is possible to move away from thinking about miasms as a "bad" thing, something that we need to be rid of; that they are instead an invitation to explore new ways of thinking, behaving and living. In other words, that miasms are an opportunity, including, as Ian suggests, for a shift in consciousness.

I love seeing examples of how these opportunities present themselves. These opportunities become especially apparent to me with two of the conventional miasms particularly. Firstly, when those with an active syphilitic miasm enter into a recovery process regarding their addictions. Secondly, when those with an active cancer miasm start to draw healthy boundaries – possibly for the first time in their lives – and do what feels good to them, rather than what feels good to everybody else. Of course not everyone with these active miasms does this, but when they do, it is a beautiful and poetic illustration of our ability as human beings to change and adapt so that we can survive, and wonderful evidence of Ian's suggestion of miasms being an opportunity.

There has been a gentle movement over time to think about miasms according to the original meaning of this concept. We have been expanding our list of miasms to include more literal "taints" or pollutants" as miasms, including the radiation and petrochemical miasms. This makes sense when we consider Dr Hahnemann's description of true, natural chronic diseases.

"The true, natural, chronic diseases are those that arise from a chronic miasm. When left to themselves (without the use of remedies that are specific against them) these diseases go on increasing. Even with the best mental and bodily dietetic conduct, they mount until the end of life, tormenting the person with greater and greater sufferings. Besides those diseases that are engendered by medical malpractice (§74), these are the most numerous and greatest tormentors of human race, in that the most robust constitution, the best regulated lifestyle, and the most vigorous energy of the life force are not in a position to eradicate them."

- Aphorism 78

Before we look further at this, I am going to take us further back – back in time to the earliest days that we have recorded of the understanding of miasms, and the true meaning of what they are.

Miasms – the early beginnings

Miasma Theory has been around for many centuries, but the understanding of, and meaning of Miasms has evolved through the ages.

The Merriam-Webster Dictionary defines miasma as:

1 : a vaporous exhalation formerly believed to cause disease

2 : an influence or atmosphere that tends to deplete or corrupt[1]

This definition remains consistent with the Ancient Greek definition of a miasm being a taint or pollution.

Vitruvius, a Roman writer, described the impact of toxic swamplands as far back as the 1st century BC: "For when the morning breezes blow toward the town at sunrise, if they bring with them mist from marshes and, mingled with the mist, the poisonous breath of creatures of the marshes to be wafted into the bodies of the inhabitants, they will make the site unhealthy."[2]

---

[1] https://www.merriam-webster.com/dictionary/miasma

[2] https://en.wikipedia.org/wiki/Miasma_theory

In Ancient Greece, people would be purified of miasma, as part of their religious practices.[3] Ancient Chinese texts describe different types of miasma[4], and miasms are recognised in Ayurvedic medicine in India, where they are likened to the three doshas, vayu, pitta and kapha.[5]

Even as recently as the early 1900s, Florence Nightingale was an advocate of Miasma Theory, ensuring that patients always had access to fresh, clean air, and was an active proponent of the adoption of sanitation as a way of preventing disease.[6]

It is understandable that our connection to, and understanding of, miasms as an important concept in health has waned since the adoption of Louis Pasteur's Germ Theory in the 1880s.

Times are changing, however. There has been an explosion in the understanding of epigenetics; inherited factors that lead to particular susceptibilities and inherited diseases. In addition to this, we are now recognising a much bigger array of miasmatic influences.

---

[3] https://mythologyfacts.weebly.com/religion-rituals-and-worship.html

[4] https://en.wikipedia.org/wiki/Miasma_theory

[5] https://www.homeopathy360.com/2018/04/24/miasm-in-the-light-of-modern-era/

[6] http://www.choleraandthethames.co.uk/cholera-in-london/cholera-in-soho/florence-nightingale/

Miasms in the Modern World

There are three types of miasms[7]:
- Inherited
- Acquired
- Planetary

In homeopathy, we are familiar with the first two.

Taking in this more comprehensive understanding of a miasm being any taint or pollution (that can lead to chronic disease), It is now widely accepted that we live in a polluted world.

Planetary miasms are a newer consideration - and describes the miasms that affect the planet as a whole, eg radiation, petrochemicals and chemtrails.

It could be said whilst many of the newer miasms are not directly physical diseases, they are still a pollution to the body, a cause of chronic disease (and can affect the DNA / genes from a more contemporary perspective) and so are miasms. This is useful to further consider in the context of Dr Hahnemann's theoretical thinking about health.

Hahnemann wrote about the cause of all disease – mental, emotional, physical and spiritual. He was influenced

---

[7] https://www.detachmenttechnique.com/atavism-miasms/

by the work of the famous German philosopher Georg Wilhelm Friedrich Hegel (1770-1831). Dr Hahnemann wasn't the only leader influenced by Hegel's teachings; the great anthroposophical leader Rudolph Steiner and Carl Jung, known as the "father of modern psychology" also were.

Hegel described how there are 4 aspects to a whole person:

* The body *Körper*
* The mind *Gemut*
* The soul *Seele* (this is where we just are who we are; our place of being)
* The spirit *Geist* (this is our connection to Source / some higher spiritual aspect). In essence this is our connection to God (or Source, or Divinity, whatever you might call the wonderful unconditional love from which we are all said to have come), or to use Sigmund Freud's psychoanalytic definition, the *superconscious*.

Dr Hahnemann described how diseases were caused by the "spiritual dynamic mistunement of the organism's life", and how, the material organism and dynamis are a unity, but that thought separates them to facilitate comprehension.

Dis-ease, therefore, is caused by the disquiet that happens when the Mind (*Gemut*) does something that isn't aligned with the Spirit (*Geist* or God, or the Superconscious); where there is a gap between the Mind and the Spirit.

In other words, our highest aspect knows what is wonderful for us and what isn't; what enables us to thrive and flourish and helps others and the world around us thrive and flourish - and what doesn't. It knows when we do wonderful things for others, and when we don't. And when we don't, even when our mind tries to justify it, some inner subconscious part of us knows and *feels* uncomfortable, and feels out of integrity. That disquiet; that *dissonance* as psychologists would describe it, creates the perfect conditions for dis-ease to set in.

Our Spirit *knows* when we act in ways that are not in alignment, so when we don't, that forms a *gap* between the Mind and the Spirit, and that GAP is where disease sets in.

When we look at the miasms, they can all be seen to be caused by a gap between what the Spirit (Geist) and Mind (Gemut) are saying. They are no longer in alignment.

So the more modern miasms – the manmade acquired and planetary miasms - could be said to be diseases of the Mind first, before they become diseases within the Body, according to this model. These miasms are an expression of what happens when we aren't living in alignment with what our Spirit (Geist) would have us do. Our

Spirit would have us act in ways that love ourselves, others and the natural world. When we disconnect from Spirit, in Hegel's terms, then we lose a connection with that quiet, gentle reminder to act with love. The voice of the Mind can become louder when this imbalance sets in; and a Mind that is fearful, yearning for power, feels insecure can take over. A gap forms between the Mind and Spirit. Miasms exist because of this gap, and this can lead to chronic dis-eases in the body.

James Tyler Kent took a moralistic view with regards to miasms, and that they were caused by "sin".

I do not take a moralistic view, like Kent did, in suggesting this. We are human, living human lives. When looking at sexually transmitted infections, for example, it could be said that we would be less likely to expose ourselves to them if we were all always 100% careful in our sexual behaviours. However we are human. We have human moments where a need and desire to connect with another transgresses any and all rational thought. Also, there are cases where diseases are spread through acts of violence, or accidents too.

As Ian Watson suggests, miasms are also an opportunity; I feel an invitation for healing - a reconnection.

In exploring these ideas, I am inviting us to consider whether the human journey of disconnection from our totality is a mechanism for inviting us to reconnect and come back to it. Almost like the beating heart, filling and expelling or the lungs breathing in and out - maybe the journey of miasms takes us from the pain of disconnection to the joy of re-connection - something we would not know without disconnection in the first place.

The Blueprint Method proposes a wonderful way forward through the huge expansion in miasmatic influences that we are exposed to. But first it feels important to give a greater context around these more modern miasms, to truly understand why we need to look at how we treat and support our patients in a new way. It's not a comfortable look, but a necessary one to understand what we can positively do – and why it is necessary.

Man-made miasms

Jos Lelieveld et al., in 2020 published research showing that in 2015, around 8.8 million people died as a consequence of air pollution. The greatest effect that air pollution had on health was related to cardiovascular diseases, which accounted for 43% of these global deaths.[8] Legal history was made in the UK in 2020 when a coroner concluded that the death of a nine-year old girl, Ella

---

[8] Cardiovascular Research, Volume 116, Issue 11, 1 September 2020, Pages 1910-1917, https://doi.org/10.1093/cvr/cvaa025

Kissi-Debrah in February 2013, included air pollution as a cause.[9]

Van Jones, a well known attorney and activist in the U.S. delivered a speech at the North Dakota Oil Pipeline protests in September 2016 where he said:

"This is as simple as I can say it: water is life, oil is death. Water is life, oil is death. That's not hyperbole. What is oil? Oil is some stuff that's been dead for millions and millions of years. Oil has been dead for 60 million years. Coal has been dead for 150 million years.

Somebody's gotta brainstorm to go and dig up a bunch of dead stuff and then burn it. Burn it in their engines, burn it in their power plants. And then they're shocked. They're shocked that having pulled death out of the ground, we now have death in the lungs of our children in the form of asthma. And we now have death on our oceans in the form of oil spills. And we now have death in the skies in the form of climate chaos. What did you think was gonna happen when you started digging up all this death? What did you think was gonna happen?

So we stand for life. Let's power a new civilization based on a living sun, based on the living wind, based on the living imagination of our children and based on the

9 https://www.theguardian.com/environment/2020/dec/16/ girls-death-contributed-to-by-air-pollution-coroner-rules-in-landmark-case

cleanliness, and the purity, and the sacredness of our water."[10]

Dr Zach Bush[11] is a "Triple A Rated" medical doctor in the US (meaning he is a specialist not just in one area of medicine, but three). He is an educator and activist, and talks extensively about the biome and virome. He also campaigns for a greater understanding of the effects of pollution, in the air, but also in the form of glyphosate in the soils. All of the profits from sales of his IonBiome[12] product, a layer of carbon from the Earth that has been scientifically proven to heal a leaky gut, go to a foundation that he created that financially supports farmers in the US as they transition from intensive farming practices to sustainable organic farming, free from the use of glyphosate and any other toxic agrochemicals. He has become an active proponent of Antoine Beauchamp's Terrain Theory, and discusses this, alongside the inaccuracies of Louis Pasteur's Germ Theory in several of his talks.

It is becoming apparent that there a recognition even in allopathic medicine and thinking that pollution causes disease, including creating changes in our genetic makeup - in other words, an acceptance of miasms – even though this term is currently only used by homeo-

---

[10] https://www.youtube.com/watch?v=L_6rSQSAl7c

[11] https://zachbushmd.com

[12] https://ionbiome.com

paths and naturopaths, and dismissed as an "obsolete medical theory" by conventional thinking.[13]

The acquired and planetary miasms being created lead us to a New Miasmatic Map.

---

[13] https://en.wikipedia.org/wiki/Miasma_theory

A New Miasmatic Map

The following Miasmatic Map evolved out of the proving of EBV conducted by the Golden Spiral Provings Collective. In the top row of the physical column of the miasmatic map, the viruses and other miasms are all manmade. All of these can trigger the naturally occurring bacteria and fungi further down the miasmatic map, and cause some to die, and others to grow more and become pathogenic – the balance and alignment between them becomes lost. Radiation and nano bots enervate all pathogens, including EBV. It is not a complete map, but it gives an indication of how big the miasmatic map has in modern times, I would suggest, become.

I would suggest that some of the man-made miasms can also activate some of the original miasms too. So I would suggest that we are moving into times we we need to be addressing   several miasms at a time, not just one.

It is necessary to look at the broad range of miasms in more detail, to understand why a newer approach to treating patients – this Blueprint Method – is needed. It's not the most comfortable realisation to have, but at the same time, there is so much hope – and a way forward……..an opportunity and an invitation that can come from understanding what follows.

Man-made / patriarchal influences

Naturally occurring

TRAUMA

Trauma as the "Mother Miasm" (Nick Biggins)

FIRST SEPARATION TRAUMA: FROM SOURCE

ANCESTRAL TRAUMA

SECOND SEPARATION TRAUMA: FROM MOTHER

SPIRITUAL

Disconnection from MEANING & NATURE as centre of life

Materialism as centre of life

Having to choose between being "scientific" (according to narrow definition of science) or religion / spiritual

mind/logic more important than heart

MENTAL

EMOTIONAL

Fear   Pressure   Stress
"Not good enough"
Fear of failure
Negative news feeds
Social media when used negatively
any "ism" (classism / racism / sexism / disables / homophobia)
financial pressure   low wages   capitalism
corporatism   social unrest
Systems that divide & conquer
(police, courts, formal education, financial)
manipulation   coercion / control
conformity   narcissism   sociopathy
psychopathy   encouragement of self-loathing
hatred of self / others
cosmetic surgery & treatments
pornography   war
Women: periods as unclean / dirty
Men: tears as weak

PHYSICAL

Manmade viruses & vibrations

HIV   COVID   Ebola   Lyme's
EBV   Radiation   Nanobots   5G

Substances

Pharmaceutical drugs
Synthetic hormones
Petrochemicals* (including plastics)
Petroleum / CO / CO2 / NO3
Teflon.   Chemtrails**
Agrochemicals & GMOs***   Heavy metals
Flouride & Chlorine   Cane sugar
Chemical drugs (eg cocaine)   Cane sugar
High fructose corn / rice syrup
Artificial sweeteners   Artificial foods

Naturally occurring pathogens

Staphylococcus aureus (including MRSA)
Streptococcus   E coli   Candida
Heliobacter pylorii   Klebsiella
Pneumococcus   Clostridium

GEOENGINEERING / MANMADE WEATHER

GAMING

CANCER

Typhoid   Leprosy   Psora   Sycotic   Syphilitic   Ringworm   Malaria   Tubercular

New Miasmatic Map
by
© Danica Apolline-Matić 2024

31

* Petrochemicals include sodium lauryl sulphate, parabens, synthetic perfumes, VOCs, flame retardants, synthetic cleaning chemicals, formaldehyde, hand sanitisers, ammonium compounds including bleach, acetaldehyde, benzene, ethylene diamine tetraacetic acid (EDTA), phthalates, polyethylene glycol (PEG) and others from the 3000+ petrochemicals that are in existence

** Agrochemicals include glyphosate, DDT, agent orange, synthetic herbicides, pesticides, fungicides

*** Heavy metals include aluminium, mercury, lead and those in chemtrails (strontium, barium, rubidium, arsenic, bromide, lithium, cadmium, the metals in the lanthanides series and others)

Trauma as the "Mother Miasm"

Nick Biggins, a brilliant homeopath and member of the Golden Spiral Provings Collective, during the proving of Petrified Sequoia, in one of his many strokes of genius, proposed that "Trauma is the "Mother Miasm".

This New Miasmatic Map embodies this principle; that all of these miasms are an expression in some way of trauma - physically, emotionally, mentally and/or spiritually - and further proposes that the single greatest cause of trauma, other than natural disasters and accidents, is the behaviour of the patriarchy.

Definition of Trauma

Trauma comes from the Greek word for wound. The inspirational doctor and world leader on trauma, Gábor Maté, describes trauma as being our woundedness or how we cope with it, that it shapes much of our behaviour, our social habits and informs our way of thinking.

There are different definitions of trauma. One of the most comprehensive definitions is this one, developed as part of the Missouri Model of Trauma Informed Care.

"Individual trauma results from an event, series of events, or set of circumstances that is experienced by an individual as physically or emotionally harmful or threatening and that can have lasting adverse effects on the individual's functioning and physical, social, emotional well-being."

I would add spiritual to that, of course, because I see us as having four levels of being physical, emotional, mental, and spiritual.

There are three main types of trauma:

Acute trauma
Chronic trauma
Complex Trauma

Acute trauma results from a single incident. So it's a one-off situation where somebody might have experienced trauma. It doesn't necessarily mean that just because it's one single incident that it's not serious, because that one single incident could be really very serious. It could be a huge naturally-occuring environmental disaster, a serious accident or an attack, for example. So acute trauma can be incredibly difficult for somebody to process.

Chronic trauma is repeated and prolonged, so happens over a period of time, such as neglect, domestic violence or abuse.

Complex trauma is exposure to varied and multiple traumatic events, often of an invasive interpersonal nature. Complex PTSD, or CPTSD, is a term used medically to describe this.

Examples of trauma include:

Sexual or physical abuse or assaults, war, oppression, natural disasters, serious accidents, traffic accidents, fires, kidnap, displacement, being a refugee, grief, starvation, famine, poverty, outbreaks of dis-ease. parental alienation, weather manipulation, political unrest, inequality, toxicity, pollution, industrial farming, petrochemicals, pharmaceuticals - just to name a few.

Aside from naturally occurring weather disasters or geo-logical events, and accidents, most traumas we see can be traced back to the actions of the patriarchy.

The First & Second Traumas

In Family Constellations work, we also consider two other traumas as the first traumas that we experience.

The first is the experience of separating from our true home; the home of our soul; our separation from Source (or God or the Divine Mother, or whatever we might wish to call the remarkable unconditional love from which we have all come).

Co-dependency - an addiction to love - which some research suggests that over 90% of us experience at some point[14], is characterised by low self-esteem, over-giving, people-pleasing, poor boundaries, controlling behaviours.

I have come to view co-dependency as an expression of the "First Trauma" - the separation from Source, and our yearning to be back "home", in that bubble of pure unconditional love.

For those that consider Source to be a feminine principle; the Divine Mother; then this is our first experience of a separation from the Mother; this is an experience wholly in the energy field.

The Second Trauma is said to be the second experience of separation from pure unconditional love that we have; it is our birth. Another separation from the Mother. Again, we experience a yearning to be with her. This is an experience that is physical, emotional, mental and spiritual.

These traumas characterise our need to be loved.

Trauma & environmental disasters

Environmental disasters can cause huge trauma. Many of us will remember the Tsunami in December 2004, which really gave us an insight into how awful such

---

[14] Cretser, G., Lombardo, W. K. (1999) Examining Codependency in a College Population College Student Journal, v33 n4 p629-37

events can be. News reports beamed 24/7 around the world really showed us the trauma of people losing their lives, losing loved ones - and worse - being unable to find their missing loved ones. People in unprecedented numbers lost their homes and their livelihoods. Such devastating consequences of environmental disasters cannot be underestimated in terms of how they affect us.

It must be noted that we are also seeing environmental disasters that are man-made. The 2024 floods in Dubai were caused by cloud seeding, and this is openly discussed in Dubai. In fact, in Dubai, people have reports - as we would have weather reports - letting people know how much cloud seeding is going on. In Dubai, it is being sold as a wonderful thing that the Government is doing to help with the heat and to combat climate change. Compensation has been immediately given to those affected by the floods, in recognition of how this was caused by the Government's actions.

Trauma & accidents

There are two aspects to consider when thinking about accidents. Firstly, was it unavoidable? Or was it caused by the neglect of a duty of care that someone else's responsible for?

For example, it may be that an accident just happened as "one of those things". I broke my wrist running around being silly with friends at University on a wet day, slipping on some wet tiles. It ended up being a situation we laughed about. However some people's bones break easily and they end up in traumatic situations as a result. For example people who accidentally shatter a leg bone, or experience a fracture of the spine, and so may need to have surgery, and may spend months in hospital and need rehabilitation - including learning how to walk again. The trauma of that can be devastating.

Trauma & the response of loved ones

How we respond to a traumatic event a loved one is experiencing can contribute to whether it becomes a traumatic event for them or not.

Research in mental health, for example, demonstrates a direct correlation between a family's immediate response when a loved one has a psychotic episode, and their ability to find their way to wellness. If a family expresses their distress at the situation openly to their loved one experiencing a psychosis, this is likely to cause a worsening of both symptoms, their loved ones' ability to recover, and is a strong predictor of a relapse. This has been found to be the case with people with schizophrenia, eating disorders and depression.[15] This response is known as expressed emotion (EE). Families that hold a steady, safe, understanding and peaceful space (even when they themselves will feel upset by the

_____

[15] Venkatasubremanian, Ganesan; Amaresha, Anekal (2012) Expressed Emotion in Schizophrenia: An Overview. Indian Journal of Psychological Medicine 34 (1) 12-20

situation) see a quicker and easier recovery in their loved one.

We saw this to great effect with the pandemic in 2020. The divide between those who took the vaccine and those who didn't was an intense experience for everyone, whichever side of the divide they were on.

For those who chose to vaccinate, they experienced huge anxieties about the fate of loved ones who chose not to, and vice versa. Families were divided, some people ostracised from their families for the choices that they made.

Which leads perfectly on to talk about the single greatest cause of trauma in our modern world.

Trauma & the patriarchy

Having mentioned trauma in relation to natural disasters and accidents, I do feel it's important to turn our focus to the main source of trauma in our times - and the main cause of miasms that we see and treat as homeopaths.

The patriarchy.

The patriarchy is a consciousness that has one modus operandi - to "divide and conquer". It does so in every way it possibly can, using fear, manipulation, coercion and control. It divides:

- nations and tribes through planting thoughts of hatred and arming both sides of conflicts around the world
- Us from nature by making a simple agricultural life seem like it is poor; creating a glitzy appeal of materialism and living in cities that poor people were told had streets lined with gold; that there is an opportunity to be "rich" with money rather than seeing the riches of the natural world, connection with our loved ones

- Us from living balanced, happy lives, where we have time to enjoy life, relax, give time, care and love to our partners, children and loved ones by making us have to work ridiculously hard and long hours just to barely survive

- Each other by seeding doubt, division and conflict within groups; pitting women and men against each other, even women against women, men against men, mothers and fathers against each other, straight people and gay people against each other, people of colour and white people against each other
- The individual from the Collective

- Us from loving ourselves and our bodies through valuing only thinness and youthfulness and portraying fat and aging as bad / ugly / unwanted

- Us from knowing who we really are, and how we express ourselves at a deep level, at our core, by seeding doubts and confusion about our gender and sexuality, or that long term monogamous relationships can bring us happiness (please note: I adore and resonate with the understanding taught in First Nation American and Canadian Indigenous Cultures that there are people with "Two Spirits"; who are transgender, and I love, honour and value that we live in a world where men can and do love men and / or women, and women can and do love men and / or women - however I feel the numbers we are seeing in the world are way beyond what we would see naturally due to hormones in the water, plastics and coercion and manipulation of young people, and the use of new trends. The confusion that ensues as a result can be really traumatic, because young people become divided from themselves, and the relationships they would naturally choose that would bring them happiness and joy. Hatred is encouraged against anyone who asks questions about the loss of balance is what we are seeing in the world)

- Us from the power and wisdom of the Divine Feminine

- Us from our creativity and the healing, transformative, awakening power of art by cutting it out of education systems designed to only celebrate knowledge, facts, logic and vocational studies

- Us from our creative thinking, by telling us what to think, rather than teaching us to question all that we are told

- Us from our intuition, by dismissing matters of the heart, gut feeling, by valuing only logic and "rational thought"

- Us from an understanding of true, natural health and the ability to be healthy by polluting our food, air and water

- Us from our health by giving us, even forcing on us at times, pharmaceutical drugs, which make us sick

- Us from the health giving properties, and activations of our pineal gland and higher consciousness, of our connection with the Sun by blocking it out using chemtrails / Solar Radiation Management (SRM) / geoengineering

- Us from wisdom by discrediting age and older people and only valuing youthfulness

- Us from spiritual practice and the Divine Mother / Source / Goddess / God

- Us from meaning and connection being at the centre of our lives, as understood by Indigenous people - by placing materialism at the centre of our lives instead

- Us from understanding what resonance is; a feeling of what feels true to us and what doesn't feel true to us. So we lose our connection to our centre

- Us from our ancestors, and an understanding that we have a soul; that there is a spiritual life, that there are angels; that there is more than this life

- Us from the truth that we are more than mere physical matter - that we have energy fields; huge, vast energy fields that extend way beyond the physical bodies we live in

All these things make us lose our *power* - individually, and as a collective. If we all felt strong enough, connected enough, unafraid enough, we would stand together and the patriarchy would cease to exist.

I would suggest that the patriarchy is an expression of what happens when we are furthest from the pure unconditional love of Source. It may also be an opportunity - an invitation - to reconnect, to heal, to return to love. That, I believe is the world we are moving into - a time beyond the patriarchy - a New Earth that is a return to love.

Ancestral Trauma

Research increasingly shows that unhealed traumas can be passed down through the DNA. We don't just inherit physical "pollutants" or miasms, we also inherit emotional, mental and spiritual "pollutants" or miasms.

This is what Family Constellations explore and, as fellow Homeopath and Constellations Facilitator Poppy Altman once shared with me, are the next stage in miasmatic theory. I wonder if Dr Hahnemann had continued to live, he may even have expanded his work on chronic diseases to include this understanding.

Slavery, or war, or the loss of a child, or any other trauma that hasn't been healed literally becomes written into the DNA, so that subsequent generations can end up expressing it.

Two examples of this really stand out for me from my experiences and work with constellations.

In the first, a mother asked for help with her teenage daughter. The mother was constantly anxious about her health, would insist on going to all her 16 year old's doctors appointments to check her daughter wasn't being given the pill or anything else the mother disagreed with. This was causing problems in the relationship because the teenage daughter wanted her privacy, and felt her mother was being overbearing. In the constellation, we saw that three generations previously, there had been a tragic accident where a child was accidentally killed by the father who had not seen the child and driven over him. The work of the constellation was to bring healing and peace to the soul of the child, and to allow those parents who had been affected to express their grief, which at the time they had not done. Their suppressed grief had become written into their DNA, and passed down until this descendant - the mother whose constellation we were witnessing - was expressing it. Releasing the suppressed grief from four generations ago brought great peace and calm to the mother.

In the second, a father asked for help with his suicidal son. In exploring the constellation, we saw that almost the entire family several generations previously had been wiped out in a war. The survivors had literally begged to be able to die to join their family. This trauma of yearning to be dead and so with their deceased loved ones had passed down until we were seeing it with the suicidal son. The constellation invited the ancestor who had survived the massacre to express their grief fully, releasing the stuck grief from the field, and easing the pressure on the son.

New Miasms that affect us physically

Before we explore more about what we can do, and what is possible for us as homeopaths using the Blueprint Method, I'd like to give clearer examples of how we are affected physically in the world, to illustrate more clearly why we now need a new way of working that transcends all that we face.

For now, I will touch on three of the miasms here: petro-chemicals, glyphosate and chemtrails, before we explore what we can do as homeopaths, and introduce the

Blueprint Method. This information is shared from *Nature's Medicine Code*[16].

Petrochemicals

Petrochemicals are used in almost every aspect of our lives; from cleaning products, to toiletries, cosmetics and perfumes, to the production of furniture and home furnishings. They are literally chemicals made using petroleum. Going back to Van Jones' description of petroleum being a substance made from death, we can start to understand why so many of these petrochemicals are linked to cancers, hormonal disturbances and a range of health conditions. The great news is that there are healthy, natural alternatives, made from "life" as Van Jones would describe; from the abundant natural world around us.

I will mention a few of these here.

Ethylene Oxide

This petrochemical is used as a sterilisation agent when steaming isn't possible. It is sprayed onto the ends of swabs used in smear tests, and on the swabs for COVID-19 tests.

---

[16] [16] Danica Apolline-Matić (2024) Nature's Medicine Code (Second Edition) Danica Apolline-Matić

It is a Class 1 Carcinogen according to the International Agency for Research on Cancer (IARC). It is also oil based, and so bioaccumulates, so there will be no safe exposure levels.

Hand Sanitisers

Research published in one of the British Medical Journals is showing a noticeable rise in thyroid cancer in people who use hand sanitisers a lot – particularly healthcare professionals, and those who . One study of over 900 patients found that women with any occupational exposure at all were 48% more likely to develop thyroid cancer, and men were 300% more likely to develop thyroid cancer.[17] We have seen an explosion in the use of these since COVID.

Parabens

Parabens are petrochemicals now well known to mimic oestrogen. They are a preservative used not just in cosmetics, creams, shaving gels and antiperspirants. Some would say that the estrogenic effect is weak, however in combination with other hormone disrupting chemicals could build up the risk. Whilst a debate about whether they cause cancer has been ongoing or over a

---

[17] Zeng F, Lerro C, Lavoué J, et al Occupational exposure to pesticides and other biocides and risk of thyroid cancer Occupational and Environmental Medicine 2017;74:502-510.

decade, they have been found in the breast cancer tissue of women with breast cancer. Breast cancers require higher levels of oestrogen to grow.

Phthalates

Dibutylphthalate is a phthalate that helps skin care to be absorbed by the skin, yet is recognized a "probable human carcinogen" by the US' Environmental Protection Agency, yet continues to be widely used by most high street cosmetic producers.

Phthlates are associated with altered DNA integrity in human sperm[18] and can affect human reproductive health.[19] So it makes it all the more concerning that phthalates are found in sex toys, as well as in skin creams. (And the good news is that some companies make phthalate-free sex toys, some companies even make them using crystals).

Perfumes

---

[18] Duty SM et al., The relationship between environmental exposures to phthalates and DNA damage in human sperm using the neutral comet assay. Environ Health Perspect. 2003 Jul;111(9):1164-9. doi: 10.1289/ehp.5756. PMID: 12842768; PMCID: PMC1241569.

[19] Hauser R, Calafat AM. Phthalates and human health. Occup Environ Med. 2005;62(11):806-818. doi:10.1136/oem.2004.017590

Perfumes contain many toxic ingredients. When you see the word "fragrance", what it really means is "hidden chemicals". Perfume and beauty product manufacturers are allowed by law to keep their fragrance ingredients secret, as trade-secret formulas.

The Campaign for Safe Cosmetics commissioned laboratory tests that found 38 chemicals not listed on the labels in 17 branded fragrances (including Chanel, Giorgio Armani, Bath & Body Works, Old Spice, Calvin Klein, and others). The average was 14 unlisted chemicals, including hormone disrupters, chemicals that are known to cause allergic reactions, diethyphthalate (found in 97% of Americans, and linked to sperm damage), and chemicals that accumulate in fat tissue and are found in breast milk.

Sodium Lauryl Sulphate

Sodium Lauryl Sulphate (SLS) is a foaming agent added in large quantities (usually the first ingredient listed) to make your cleansing product feel as though its foam is making you clean.

Polyethylene Glycols

Polyethylene Glycols (PEG) are moisturisers, stabilisers and solvents that make a more consistent product. It is found in moisturisers, creams, cleansers and lots of baby products. They are often contaminated with pollutants including ethylene oxide, dioxane, polycyclic aromatic compounds and heavy metals including arsenic, cadmium, lead, nickel, cobalt and iron. This increases skin permeability and allows pollutants to enter the body through the skin's surface. Dermatitis and irritation are common effects of PEGs. The contaminants often found in PEGs are known carcinogens. Specifically, they have been linked to breast cancer, leukaemia, brain and nervous system cancer, bladder cancer, stomach cancer and pancreatic cancer, as well as Hodgkin's disease. They have been proven to interfere with development, especially the nervous system, and may cause kidney and liver organ toxicity.

Flame Retardants

Most mattresses and sofas, car seats, curtains and upholstered furniture proudly display that they meet legal safety standards to be flame retardant. However these are the most toxic substances we can bring into our home. Brominated flame retardants have been linked to a range of health problems and diseases including infertility, birth defects, behavioural problems in children, and liver, kidney, testicular and breast cancers and autoimmune disorders. Because they are fat soluble, they accumulate in the fat in the body, including in breast tissue, and are found in breast milk.

Formaldehyde, a known carcinogen used to preserve dead bodies, is found in most flat-pack furniture, often in the adhesives used in composite wood products such as particle board, fiberboard and plywood.

The good news is that there are natural alternatives; wool is naturally flame retardant and so wool mattresses and sofas don't have to be sprayed with these chemicals.

This is particularly concerning given that a 2004 study found more than 200 chemicals such as these in the umbilical cords of babies.[20]

Petroleum Jelly

We think that reaching out for our tub of Vaseline or aqueous cream is just the best thing to do when we have dry lips or skin.

Have you ever thought why petroleum jelly is called petroleum jelly? I didn't. For years. Then it hit me. It is a jelly made from petroleum. You know, the substance we make petrol from. The ingredient made from dead dinosaurs I mentioned above? That known carcinogen we have just been talking about? All smeared all over your lips and skin, waiting to go into your body.

Urgh no. I don't think so. There are amazing vegan, organic, 100% natural alternatives that work brilliantly. Or indeed we can learn to make our own!

---

[20] https://www.ewg.org/research/body-burden-pollution-newborns

Teflon

In the UK, every school uniform comes coated in Teflon or other stain repellant / non-stick coating, that is a carcinogen. Teflon is said to be carcinogenic only at high temperatures but it doesn't break down in the environment, and when children get hot and sweaty, there aren't any guarantees that some of the coating isn't entering the body. Also, the US has decided to restrict the use of a chemical used in the manufacture of Teflon......any alarm bells ringing yet?

This is a classic example of where many of us aren't erring on the side of caution.......but these are our precious children.

In the UK, the only way to buy uniform that is NOT coated in Teflon or any other stain repellant or non-stick coating is to buy organic uniform, which isn't in everyone's price range. It means you have to iron the uniforms, but at least the uniform is a healthy one.

For the time my son had to wear uniform, I refused to buy him the standard issue uniform with the school logo badge on the sweater, and told the school why. The staff there loved me as was clear from the rolling of their eyes. But we have to do this as parents. Make a stand. You are a powerful voice and consumer. Demand your child's school provides other options that are not coated in synthetic (and in this toxic) chemicals, and talk to other parents about this issue and get them on board.

In the UK, Eco Outfitters is a great company for organic school uniforms.

Glyphosate

Kate Birch's excellent book Glyphosate Free[21] describes what glyphosate does at a biochemical level in the body, before describing how we can detox ourselves and our patients.

Glyphosate sits in the receptor sites that would normally be occupied by the amino acid glycine. Glycine is the simplest of all the amino acids, and can be obtained through food and made by the body. It is used to make vitamin B9 (folate), tryptophan, serotonin and melatonin, and is needed for cardiovascular processes and immunity. Glycine is needed for the production of adenine, which is converted to adenosine (and used to make adenosine triphosphate – ATP; energy generated in our mitochondria). It is also needed to make phenylananine, a precursor for tyrosine which is used to make dopamine and other neurotransmitters, T3 and T4. Glycine is also important in the body's natural detoxification process.

---

[21] Kate Birch (2019) Glyphosate Free: An Essay on Functional Nutrition and the Homeopathic Clearing of Glyphosate Toxicity Kate Birch

Because glyphosate sits in the glycine receptor sites, it interrupts all of the processes that use glycine.

Glyphosate is everywhere; in our air, and soils. However as well as clearing glyphosate homeopathically, trying our best to eat only organic foods where possible to reduce exposure to glyphosate helps not just us but the world around us.

Chemtrails

There are three interesting features of chemtrails. Firstly, the use of radioactive elements (strontium and barium). Secondly, the use of lithium, which is a mood stabiliser that suppresses extremes of emotion (extremes of emotion which could ignite revolutions? the interesting features of chemtrails, which contribute to air pollution, is that they include the lanthanides series of metals.

As homeopathic remedies, the lanthanides were discovered by Dr Jan Scholten, MD, and Magister Robert Münz. Jan is a homoeopathic doctor with a chemistry background, and Robert is a homoeopathic pharmacist.

Jan Scholten's book The Secret Lanthanides[22] interestingly makes the link with the Greek word for self

---

[22] Jan Scholten (2005) The Secret Lanthanides Stichting Alonnissos, Utrecht

"autos" which is linked to one of the ways in which Lanthanides are used; for treating auto-immune diseases, and the other feature of the picture with Lanthanides; that individuals seek autonomy; to be in control of themselves and their own lives.

Autonomy is considered to be a core keyword for Lanthanides. Jan states that "Lanthanides desire freedom, liberty, independence and being their own boss. They want to lead their own life. Self-determination is essential. They can look like anarchists. They cannot stand being dominated, dictated to, being taken over, manipulated and ruled. They have a strong aversion to doctors, operations and injections. It feels for them a violation of their own integrity."

What is interesting about Lanthanides, as Jan describes, is that they don't want autonomy – and the freedom that goes with it – for themselves, but for others also. Because of this, they tend to be humanists, wanting everyone to be free and independent.

This leads me to wonder whether lanthanides therefore, in material form, bring with them some sense of control; of controlling others, preventing them from being autonomous.

Applying The New Miasmatic Map

Looking at this new map, two understandings become clear. Firstly, almost all of it is man-made. The explosion in pollutants – miasma – has occurred due to human influence over the last 150 years, and has completely transformed our exposure to pollutants since Dr Samuel Hahnemann's time.

Secondly, if we were only to work miasmatically or using tautopathy, to clear the effects of the man-made pollutants on the being, we would probably be working well beyond one lifetime, especially when we consider that there are over 3,000 petrochemicals alone!

I would like to propose that working miasmatically, and using detoxification protocols are still of vital importance to us as homeopaths, but that we need a bit more help with supporting the vital force of our patients to clear the effects of all that they face.

We need to go higher than the physical challenges we face, transcending these, by working with the fundamentals of who and, more importantly, what we are.

Energy beings.

This is where the Blueprint Method comes in. Before I explain what it is, and the remedies that make up the Blueprint Method, I will take us back to a re-visit of how we are made; of what we are.

The following is another excerpt from *Nature's Medicine Code*.[23]

---

[23] Danica Apolline-Matić (2024) Nature's Medicine Code (Second Edition) Danica Apolline-Matić

A Sojourn into Science

You may think of yourself as solid, dense, physical matter, but actually all of us are mainly made up of space. This is how.

We are physically made up of atoms. They look like this.

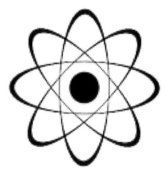

The physical matter of an atom is its nucleus – that bit in the centre – the rest surrounding it is energy. That physical matter in an atom only accounts for 1% of the atom - the other 99% is space - or energy. So that means that you, as something made of atoms, is therefore 1% physical matter and 99% space.

Marcus Chown in his book *Quantum Theory Cannot Hurt You,* gives the amazing statistic that, if all of the space within atoms and between atoms was removed, 99.99% of the entire population of the world – 99.99% of over 7 billion of us – would fit into the size of a sugar cube. Amazing, isn't it?!

So what is that space filled with? It is filled with energy.

How do we know there is this pool of energy? Dogs can hear sounds that we can't hear. Infrared light is a light frequency that we can't see with our physical eyes, but science measures sound frequencies and light frequencies that we as humans can't experience with our physical bodies. These frequencies are an expression of energy. So there is so much energy – so many frequency vibrations – that we don't experience physically but that we can measure and so know exist. The world is made of more than we can physically sense. These frequencies that we can't see or hear don't just exist outside of ourselves, they exist within us too.

Your thoughts, your feelings and your beliefs live in the energy within and around you. When you feel a little bit sick about something you know you have to do, but don't want to, you might feel it in your body a bit, but there isn't an organ that we can measure that says "this is the bit where dread lives". But we feel dread within us, and just outside of our physical bodies – dread is a feeling that we often sense in the air directly in front of our stomach. The same is true of "butterflies in our stomach". We feel these not just within our stomachs, but we can feel it in the space and the air in front of our bodies. The same happens with joy. We can't *measure* it in our bodies, but we might feel light as a feather, a lightness *within and around* us. Our feelings – and our thoughts - exist but are not contained within any one body system. That is because they don't live there. They live in the vast amounts of *space* that I have described, the 99% that isn't physical matter. In other words, our thoughts, feelings and beliefs are part of the energy within and around us.

This space – this energy – is known as the electromagnetic field, as is being studied by the HeartMath Institute in the U.S. It has measured that the electromagnetic field extends to up to 20ft from the heart.

The space within us and the space around us is filled with the energy made by a vast number of tiny light particles – they are called photons. Photons are the smallest quantum particles we know (mega tiny compared to atoms). We all have the same energy within and around us – this is the energy that quantum physicists study.

This is how, to quote Albert Einstein "everything is energy". Einstein, Nikola Tesla and Isaac Newton (after his work on gravity), three of the greatest scientists who ever lived were fascinated by energy, by quantum physics, by an understanding that we are more – much more – than physical matter.

Our Energy Field as a Sarcode

We have been taught that our largest organ is the skin.

An organ is defined as: "a part of an organism which is typically self-contained and has a specific vital function".

On this basis, I propose that our largest organ is NOT our skin. It is our *energy field*.

The 99% of us affected by trauma is an organ that also needs support, healing and remedies.

Trauma & the energy field

What would happen if we use remedies that take us right back to what our blueprint - our energy field; the 99% of us - looks like when it's whole?

What happens when we use remedies that are about the sacred geometry and the Phi mathematics, the vibration of love with which we have been created?

What if we have access to, and use, a new generation of sarcode remedies - organ remedies for our true largest organ - our energy field?

Trauma affects our geometry, as we understand from the work of Dr. Masuro Emoto and now Veda Austin.

Dr Masuro Emoto proved to us, through photographing ice formed from water carrying different vibrations, that our thoughts, feelings and intentions can literally heal or harm by altering the natural geometry in water. 60-75% of us is made of water.

Dr Masuro Emoto showed us that when we are connected with the vibration of love which, according to Manfred Clynes, is the expression of Phi mathematics - 1.618, the geometry is water is perfect and beautiful. Love generates this perfect geometry - which makes us whole at a cellular level, and also at an energetic level.

When we're surrounded by messages of hate and when we're surrounded by trauma, doubt, self-doubt, gaslighting, all that goes on in the world, then we lose our geometry, we lose our integrity, we lose our wholeness.

The geometry of our energy field

When we look at the Flower of Life, it contains all the other sacred geometry. It contains within it the Golden Spiral, the Seed of Life, the Egg of Life, the Fruit of Life, the Tree of Life and more.

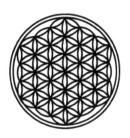

I am going to briefly describe what these all represent, because when we understand what they all represent, we understand the aspects of life that become difficult for us to access when our geometry is compromised, when we are being affected by trauma.

When the Flower of Life is compromised and no longer the shape of the Flower of Life, deformed by trauma, then we can't access all that the Flower of Life represents. And when the Flower of Life is deformed, we also can't access the geometry we find within it - we can't access the Golden Spiral, the Seed of Life, the Egg of Life, the Fruit of Life, the Tree of Life and all that these do for us in our journey through life. What follows is a summary of each of these component geometric shapes. More information can be found at Rare Earth Gallery.[24]

---

[24] https://www.rareearthgallerycc.com/blog-entry/91/intro-duction-to-sacred-geometry

The Seed of Life is, very simply, how life starts from a seed and then blossoms and grows. That's what it represents. It connects us with blessings, with protection, with creation.

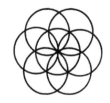

The Egg of Life is an expression of the stage of growth of an embryo when it's divided into four and then it moves into eight cells, we see the egg of life. The Egg of Life represents health, stability and fertility.

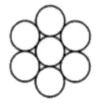

The Fruit of Life is made of 13 spheres, and 13 is a number of unity and connection through dimensions and worlds. It's also the number of the Sacred Feminine. We have 13 lunar cycles, 13 moon cycles in any calendar year. So, of course, the patriarchy has done a wonderful job of making us think the number 13 is unlucky, so we don't connect with actually how powerful a number it is. And 13 comes down to the four, which is about stability and at its foundation. So, we've got the fruit of life connecting us with the Sacred Feminine; with our ability to materialise - to welcome into physical matter that which is in spirit. To literally turn our dreams into our reality. The Fruit of Life also connects us with unity and presence.

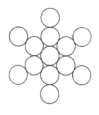

The Tree of Life is found in the Kabbalah, and is geometrically also found within the Flower of Life. It is made of 11 Sephirot, or aspects of life that connect us with our journey or path to God (Source). The Sephirot include knowledge, wisdom, connection, healthy boundaries, love and kindness, sovereignty, our ability to materialise to manifest, and the vibration of victory as well.

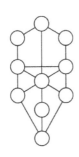

Within the Flower of Life we also have the Grid of Life, which is made of 64 tetrahedrons. The Grid of Life connects us with our soul or star family, and all that we have agreed to complete in our lives together collectively. The Grid of Life realigns us with them and our collective goals, so that we can manifest or materialise our desires and dreams more easily.

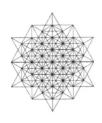

The Merkabah is also found within the Flower of Life. It is made of two intersecting tetrahedrons. We've got the masculine pointing up and the feminine pointing down. And basically, this is what our aura looks like when it's stationary. When the Merkabah is spinning in a healthy way, then what happens is that each tetrahedron is going in an opposite direction to the other to generate an incredible energetic field. It gives us power-

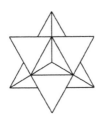

ful protection and it connects and aligns us with our higher consciousness.

The Torus is, in effect, our aura; our energy field when it's whole and complete and spinning and moving. The Torus gives us alignment and wholeness. When our Torus has been affected and isn't in alignment, we start losing our connection to love. We can start to lose empathy, and step closer towards psychopathy.

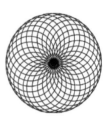

Vector Equilibrium is another geometric shape found within the Flower of Life. It connects us with moving to a point of stillness; from duality to oneness.

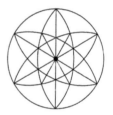

The Flower of Life is made up of all of these geometric symbols - and all that they represent.

When we think about how trauma can affect us, if trauma affects us at a geometric level - at a Flower of Life level - and alters the geometry of our energy field -, then all of the other sacred geometry that we find in the Flower of Life becomes affected.

So when we lose the integrity of the Flower of Life due to trauma - caused by all of the influences listed in the New

Miasmatic Map proposed in this book - we also lose our connection to:

- The alignment that the Golden Spiral brings, and the geometry and integrity of the DNA, our chakras, the symmetry of our bodies, the flow of blood through our bodies, alignment with our path through life
- The blessings, protection and connection with creation that the Seed of Life welcomes to us
- The health, stability and fertility that the Egg of Life connects us with
- Our connection with the Sacred or Divine Feminine, unity and presence that the Fruit of Life brings us
- All that the Tree of Life connects us with: knowledge, wisdom, connection, healthy boundaries, love and kindness, sovereignty, our ability to materialise to manifest, and the vibration of victory
- The balance, protection and alignment with our higher consciousness that the Merkabah brings us
- The connection to love, empathy, wholeness, alignment that the Torus brings us; our ability to relate to others from a loving, unified, respectful and balanced space
- The ability to experience true peace, stillness and oneness that Vector Equilibrium brings us

So in other words, trauma blocks us from all these aspects within ourselves that our geometric make up - our blueprint - can help us to experience when healthy and whole:

- Alignment, in how our body works, in how we feel and think
- Alignment with meaning & spiritual practice
- Receiving blessings
- Feeling safe and protected
- Our creativity
- Health
- Stability
- Balance
- Fertility
- Unity
- Presence
- Our ability to manifest / materialise
- Knowledge
- Wisdom
- Connection
- Healthy boundaries
- Love
- Kindness
- Sovereignty
- Victory (Success)
- Personal power
- Clarity
- A balance of masculine and feminine - and the ability to connect with both of those aspects within us in a healthy, unified, integrated way

- Alignment with our higher consciousness
- Respect
- Love
- Empathy
- Wholeness
- Strength
- Peace
- Stillness
- Oneness
- Support from others
- Alignment with soul purpose
- Connection with Source / God

Whilst the word happiness hasn't been used here, it is a given that being able to live life aligned with all of this ultimately brings us happiness.

This is our natural, healthy, healed state. These are our ways of living and being when we are whole. This is what becomes compromised through trauma. So, this is why I've started to talk about the Blueprint Method, as an addition to all of the other wonderful methods of prescribing that we have.

The Blueprint Method

What is our Blueprint, according to this Method?

The Blueprint Method uses remedies that connect us with energy vibrations of who we are when we are whole using the geometry and mathematics found in DNA, colour remedies, sound remedies, the 27 tissue salts, and remedies that reconnect us with our astrology; like organ support remedies remind our organs of what a healthy organ looks like and functions as......Blueprint Method remedies remind us of what we look like and function like when healthy and whole as a whole energetic being.

They are the new sarcodes; a new similimum; working with our energy body in its entirety.

It was James Compton-Burnett who made the connection that we can apply the law of similars to prescribing organ remedies - *like cures like* by giving remedies that speak to the organ that needs healing.

The Blueprint Method brings us back to alignment by reconnecting us with, in Hegel's terms, our "Spirit" – that part of us that is really who we are. An expression of the Divine Mother, the Goddess, God, or Source, or some higher principle. An expression of Phi Mathematics, and colour and sound vibrations. An expression of love. A re-connection with love, and the healing of the First & Second Traumas, as well as the effects of traumas caused by man.

Isn't this the same as constitutional prescribing?

This is a similar principle to prescribing constitutionally – but isn't the same. When we choose constitutional remedies, we are choosing remedies that reflect the personality of the individual. These are expressed, using Hegel's terms Mind and Soul. But who we really are beyond the human personality is Spirit (God). Spirit transcends personalities, and is an expression of pure unconditional love.

However what is similar is the effect. In essence, working constitutionally reminds us of who we are so that we, more aligned with ourselves, with a strengthened vital force, can heal – but it does so at the level of the personality.

Working at the level of the Spirit also reminds us of who are so that we, more aligned with ourselves, with a strengthened vital force, can heal. This time, it does so at the level beyond the personality; to a higher understand ing and experience of ourselves as one with Source. It's a transcendence of the human experience.

The personality might be who we are choosing to be in this lifetime, but Spirit is who and what we really are.

Why call this the Blueprint rather than Spirit Method?

In Hegel's description of the totality of a person, the Soul could be said to be linked to our personality; our place of being. Some of us would call Spirit – the connection to Source / pure unconditional love / pure energy – the soul, and would call spirit those energies that have passed into the next life.

This is why I am using the Blueprint, so that we can all be clear about what we are discussing – the who and what we really are, beyond our minds, or our personalities; our connecting to being spiritual beings, an energy, connected to Source.

The Blueprint Method adds a remedy to any prescription that aligns us with Spirit, so that we are prescribing with the totality of the individual, helping us to transcend the challenges of modern times, or inherited traumas, so that the vital force, or dynamis, is strengthened through a reconnection with Source as well as working on the other layers.

The New Miasms as an Opportunity

So we return to Ian Watson's invitation to explore new ways of thinking, behaving and living. We reconnect with Ian's assertion that miasms are an opportunity, including, as he suggests, for a shift in consciousness.

I propose that it is time for us, as homeopaths, to experience our own shift in consciousness.

We began our journey with Dr Hahnemann using homeopathy to treat dis-ease within the body. Over time, this was expanded into using homeopathy to treat dis-eases of the mind as well as the body. Now it is time for us to expand our practice to also incorporate the soul - and, in Hegel's terminology - spirit, too.

We have an opportunity to transcend the actions of the patriarchy and bring a return to wholeness for the whole being; to work with remedies that activate healing for the construct - or organ - that is our energy field; the 99% of what we truly are.

Our energy field is an expression of the mathematics of life; of sacred geometry; which is an expression of sound and vibration.

So it is time to work with remedies that are sarcodes for our biggest organ - the organ that is our energy field; our blueprint.

This enables us to transcend the influences of all of the modern man-made miasms that we find.

What is the difference between detoxing & miasmatic work?

Both detoxing & miasmatic work are, in essence, healing the vital force through the application of the Law of Similars.

Traditionally, miasmatic work is undertaken using remedies made from disease material (sarcodes). Detoxification is carried out using remedies made from a toxin (tautopathy) and remedies made from healthy organs. (sarcodes).

The Miasmatic Map has expanded so that it no longer just includes disease processes that cause dis-ease, but also toxins that cause dis-ease.

Therefore, how we treat miasms now also needs to expand to include the use of tautopathy and sarcodes.

When can we use the Blueprint Method?

We can use this method:

- When we see patients with mental health problems, repeating patterns of behaviours or situations that are challenging, or addictions. These might be caused by inherited or this-life traumas, or unclear energy fields
- When we see chronic diseases that we are having difficulties treating, especially autoimmune conditions including allergies
- With patients who are highly medicated
- With patients who were highly medicated in the past
- With those who have been affected by any of these man-made pollutants
- Those with poor self-esteem
- People who are stuck, finding it hard to find a way through life
- When doing any detoxification process
- Acute diseases like colds and flus that have a strange or unusual quality to them

I would also suggest that all of us would benefit from prophylactic work with the Blueprint Method, due to the level of influence and exposure that we have to man made influences, eg radiation, glyphosate and chemtrails.

Remedies that heal our Blueprint

Remedies that heal our blueprint include those that connect us with the geometry and Phi mathematics (of love) found in DNA, colour remedies, sound remedies, and remedies that reconnect us with our astrology (our life map).

Blueprint Method remedies remind us of what we look like and function like when healthy and whole as a whole energetic being.

Some of these have been triturated to between 12c and 28c before being made into higher potencies, according to the amazing discovery of Dr Paul Theriault and his colleague Kim Kalina.

Triturated Remedies

Triturating remedies up to c28 sends the energy of the remedy through different layers of consciousness, as mapped out by Dr Paul Theriault and Kim Kalina.

Trituration – the process of making remedies that Dr Hahnemann described – involves mixing, grinding and scraping a substance in a pestle and mortar for an hour at a time for each increase in potency. Trituration usually stops at 2c or 3c before remedies are potentised ("run up") from there.

The Trituration Handbook: into the heart of Homeopathy by Anneke Hogeland and Judy Shriebman[25] describes how triturating up to c4 takes a remedy through all of the layers of a person – physically, emotionally, mentally & spiritually.

Dr Theriault, in his brilliant book *Resurrection of the Vital Force: Blockages to Healing in Homeopathy,* describes what he discovered in his work with the homeopath Kim Kalina in terms of what happens when triturating up to c28 before potentising from there. What they found was that we send the vitality of the remedy beyond the individual, into the collective, through family systems, miasms, ancestral patterns, countries, civilisations, the planet, the solar system, galaxies, Universe all the way to The Divine at 28c.

Say a remedy has been triturated to 12c before being made into higher potencies. That means it has been triturated through the 4 layers of individual consciousness (physical - 1c, emotional - 2c, mental - 3c, spiritual - 4c), then through the family, cultural and collective layers (5c-8c), and through the layers of consciousness for our beautiful planet (9c–12c). When we take, say, a 1M potency of that remedy, we are working at the 1M potency and the remedy is working through all of

[25]Anneke Hogeland and Judy Shriebman (2008) The Trituration Handbook: into the Heart of Homeopathy HomeopathyWest

our layers, our family, our culture, the collection, and our planet. So our families and the world receives some of the healing we are experiencing too.

We are in such a profound time of transformation, evolution and expansion, and the remedies we are making reflect this through the collective. Using this method of remedy making is deeply resonant with the work we are doing.

For more information about this remarkable and deep work, please find a reference to Dr Theriault's book.[26]

All of these remedies are ONLY available at:

Stellar Online (UK & EU)
Eugenie Kruger's Shop (Australia)
PS11 (US)

An early and less vital version of Golden Spiral is available at Helios, Ainsworths and Martin & Pleasance, however I would recommend only sourcing this remedy from one of the dispensaries above, because the version they have has been triturated to a 12c according to the teachings of Dr Paul Theriault before being made to higher potencies, and so is a much more vital version of the remedy.

---

[26]Dr Paul Anderson Theriault (2019) Resurrection of the Vital Force: Blockages to Healing in Homeopath. Lulu Publishing

1) The Golden Spiral

This new remedy, first made during the Winter Solstice in December 2020 and proved in January 2021 by the Golden Spiral Provings Collective, is a remedy that is an expression of the perfect mathematical and geometric spiral found in all of nature and life, including:

- In the famous nautilus
- In the proportions of our ears, how they grow and unfold
- The arrangement of faces, in particular the positioning of our mouth and nose along with our eyes and chin
- The proportions of the uterus
- In the spirals of the DNA
- In the growth and unfolding of leaves
- The number of petals a flower has
- The arrangement of seed heads, for example clearly seen in the sunflower
- The way in which branches on trees grow or split
- Animal bodies, including starfish, ants, honeybees, and the fins on dolphins
- How hurricanes and tornados travel
- How currents flow in seas and oceans
- In the formation of ice crystals and snowflakes
- The Aurora Borealis (Northern Lights)
- How planets in our solar system orbit each other as they travel through the galaxy

- In how electrons flow around the nucleus of an atom[27]
- How the energy of balanced, healthy chakras flow

This remedy brings alignment in all it's forms, moving through blocks and barriers or unhealed past traumas in order that the alignment of the whole person from the DNA through to the higher spiritual aspect can be re-established.

It also brings an alignment with purpose, flow, a freedom from constraints and limitations, supporting the person through transitions, bring peace, calm and acceptance, strength and resilience and connection. The spiral expands as it moves; and the same is true of this remedy. It brings expansion.

It is an excellent transition remedy, and we have a case where it has pulled someone back into life from the brink of death.

This remedy can be taken in the Fibonacci potencies, as the Fibonacci sequence generates the Golden Spiral.

The proving group found that taking this remedy at a lower potency – 30c daily, is a lovely place from which to work, as the Spiral unfolds through all the other potencies above it.

---

[27] Winter,D, Donavan, B., and Jones, M. (2012) Compressions, The Hydrogen Atom and Phase Conjugation

Recently, perhaps because we are all evolving, we have been finding that working with higher potencies can also be helpful. 1M daily can be helpful if some's vital force can take it, and they are particularly stuck.

Also, there is a beautiful detoxifying combination of Golden Spiral, Flower of Life, Thuja and Silica 30c, which works to clear many toxins, including the latest vaccines. This can be taken one three times a day for 5-7 days then one daily for another 21 days.

This combination can also be used as the Saturday remedy when using Ton Jansen's detox protocols.

2) Flower of Life

This remedy, was proved in November 2023 by the Golden Spiral Provings Collective. It is a remedy that is an expression of all of the mathematics and geometry found in all of existence and life. It contains the Golden Spiral and all other sacred geometry relevant to life.

Key themes include:

- Expansion
- Light
- Activations including DNA & pineal gland & brain activations (Eye of Horus)

- Multidimensional – goes through portals of time & space
- Higher consciousness & awakening
- War trauma (including physical effects)
- Grief & sadness (heart healing, compares with Thymus Gland & Green)
- Anger (with grief - more ignatia than causticum)
- Anxiety & self-consciousness
- Clears darkness
- Gives us an overview of life (birds), reminds us of the smallness of us & our lives on this one planet travelling through the cosmos filled with billions of stars & planets
- Brings peace
- Truth is revealed easily so that healing can occur
- Opens to gratitude for life & the smallest things within me
- Energising
- It's a remedy that brings magic, abundance
- Heals relationships; connects, brings support, soul connections, being taken care of, clears those where there isn't resonance or respect
- Reminds us of our worth & value
- Makes life easier, brings more spaciousness
- Transcends the patriarchy /shows new ways to live & be that are about community & connection – brings freedom & release
- Protects the soul
- Activates the spine
- Big blood remedy
- This is a remedy about LIFE

3) Seed of Life

This is an as yet unproved remedy - to be triturated.

The Seed of Life, however, connects us with how life starts from a seed and then blossoms and grows. That's what it represents. It connects us with blessings, with protection, with creation.

4) Egg of Life

This is an as yet unproved remedy - to be triturated.

The Egg of Life is an expression of the stage of growth of an embryo when it's divided into four and then it moves into eight cells, we see the egg of life. The Egg of Life represents health, stability and fertility.

5) Fruit of Life

This is an as yet unproved remedy - to be triturated.

The Fruit of Life is made of 13 spheres, and 13 is a number of unity and connection through dimensions and worlds. It's also the number of the Sacred Feminine. We have 13 lunar cycles, 13 moon cycles in any calendar year. So, of course, the patriarchy has done a wonderful job of making us think the number 13 is unlucky, so we don't connect with actually how powerful a number it is. And 13 comes down to the four, which is about stability and at its foundation. So, we've got the fruit of life connecting us with the Sacred Feminine; with our ability to materialise - to welcome into physical matter that which is in spirit. To literally turn our dreams into our reality. The Fruit of Life also connects us with unity and presence.

6) Tree of Life

This is a remedy proved by trituration.

The Tree of Life is found in the Kabbalah, and is geometrically also found within the Flower of Life. It is made of 11 Sephirot, which are the circles in the image, or aspects of life that connect us with our journey or path to God (Source). The Sephirot include:

Malkut - sovereignty & manifestation
Yesod - foundation
Hod - surrender
Netzach - victory
Tiferet - harmony & beauty
Gemurah - strength of boundaries
Chesed - loving & kindness (unbounded love)
Da'at - knowledge (this can be hidden)
Binah - understanding
Chochmah - wisdom
Keter - crown (closest to Source/God - faith, pleasure, will)

The Tree of Life represents all that is masculine and feminine, and brings balance to both.

Key themes include:

- Holding powerful, empowered boundaries
- Brings light
- Connects us with wisdom
- Welcomes strong foundations
- Completeness
- Wholeness
- Strength
- Protection
- Balances masculine / feminine
- A sense of peace - like things will work out

7) Grid of Life

This is an as yet unproved remedy - to be triturated.

Within the Flower of Life we also have the Grid of Life, which is made of 64 tetrahedrons. The Grid of Life connects us with our soul or star family, and all that we have agreed to complete in our lives together collectively. The Grid of Life realigns us with them and our collective goals, so that we can manifest or materialise our desires and dreams more easily.

8) Merkabah

This is an as yet unproved remedy - to be triturated.

The Merkabah is also found within the Flower of Life. It is made of two intersecting tetrahedrons. We've got the masculine pointing up and the feminine pointing down. And basically, this is what our aura looks like when it's stationary. When the Merkabah is spinning in a healthy way, then what happens is that each tetrahedron is going in an opposite direction to the other to generate an incredible energetic field. It gives us powerful protection and it connects and aligns us with our higher consciousness.

9) Torus

This is an as yet unproved remedy - to be triturated.

The Torus is, in effect, our aura; our energy field when it's whole and complete and spinning and moving. The Torus gives us alignment and wholeness. When our Torus has been affected and isn't in alignment, we start losing our connection to love. We can start to lose empathy, and step closer towards psychopathy.

10) Vector Equilibrium

This is an as yet unproved remedy - to be triturated.

Vector Equilibrium is another geometric shape found within the Flower of Life. It connects us with moving to a point of stillness; from duality to oneness.

11) Petrified Sequoia

This remedy has been triturated to 28c, according to Dr Paul Theriault's teachings. This remedy was proved in 2023.

Key themes:

- Ancestral, past life & personal trauma
- Integrating split parts of ourselves / soul retrieval
- Truth - Consciousness, Awakening & Realisation
- Activism and speaking up
- From stuckness to a fresh start – a reset
- Separation, Belonging & peace
- Healing of past relationships
- Home
- Time
- Magnetic – from polarisation to centredness
- Grounding
- Depression
- Oppression

- Anxiety
- Feeling wrong and making mistakes
- Adrenal fatigue
- Birds
- Freedom

12) Welwitschia mirabilis

This is a remedy that was made and proved through trituration by Dr Paul Theriault and Michal Yakir.[28]

Welwitschia is a remarkable and one of the rarest plants in the world that only produces two (large) leaves throughout it's entire life, growing continuously along the ground. The leaves can split into many segments, due to the effect of the wind whipping the leaves. It can live for between 400 and nearly 2000 years, with separate male and female plants. It is found in Namibia, along the coastal band of the Namib desert. The San call it "the plant that can never die."

Key themes include:

- Very poor immunity
- Many infections
- Swallowing disorders
- Mould toxicity

---

[28] Dr Paul Theriault (2024) Welwitschia mirabilis seed: Death, Rebirth and Resurrection - Lulu

- Fungal colonisation
- Sense of decay and decomposition of the body, even though alive
- Osteoporosis
- Sepsis
- Waiting to die due to severe infection, but not a lot of notable outward symptoms (eg pain or distress)
- Palliative situations
- Dementia
- Needing to be in a group, but somehow finding themselves to be alone
- Conflicts
- Being stuck
- Sensitivity to rude or rough people
- Division
- Loneliness
- Reclaiming fragmented parts of the self

This remedy can move people from dying to living, finding a way back to a state of purpose once more (like Golden Spiral).

Paul and Michal found that a healthy healing of miasmatic influences, and freedom from karmic states started at 36c.

13) 9/11 Survivor Tree

This is a remedy made from a sample of the one tree that survived 9/11, collected by Hilery Dorrian and Maggie Dixon.

The tree is a Callery pear tree. Pyrus calleryana is a species of ornamental pear tree that is native to China and Vietnam. It is known for having an offensive odour. It is now found widely across the United States, having been brought over in the early 1900s. It grows easily and quickly to 30-40 ft tall in only 8-10 years, and is easy to care for, resistant to many insects, fires and diseases so is popular with homeowners.

There is a strength and determination in this tree, that it will grow no matter what is thrown at it, hence it was found still growing after 9/11. In the proving carried out by the Golden Spiral Provings Collective, there was a very strong sense of there being a forcefield, a strong and robust energetic shield that created an invincibility. Also, that this is a useful remedy to counter the effects of the patriarchy.

Key themes include:

- Survival, protection & invincibility – a forcefield
- Apocalyptic devastation to hope
- Energy and radiation
- Nothingness
- Confusion

- Resistance to fire
- Feminine Power
- Whales
- Support
- Structure
- New Beginnings
- Fertility & pregnancy
- Detoxification
- Acute hearing
- Insect Repellent

14) Sound remedies (especially the Solfeggio frequencies)

We are 99% energy, and energy is expressed as sound and colour, even if in sound frequencies we can't hear (but dogs can!) or we can't see in the visual spectrum (such as infra red).

The Ancient Solfeggio Frequencies are musical tones that make up the ancient 6-tone scale thought to have been used in sacred music, including the beautiful Byzantian or Gregorian Chants. Originally said to have been developed by a Benedictine monk, Guido d'Arezzo (c. 991 AD – c. 1050 AD), the chants and their special tones were believed to impart spiritual blessings when sung in harmony.

Each Solfeggio tone is comprised of a frequency required to balance our energy and keep our body, mind and spirit in perfect harmony.

The tones were hidden until they were rediscovered by Dr Joseph Puleo in 1974. He applied a Pythagorean method to calculating the frequencies, and then discovered a further 3 tones.

Nikola Tesla, the quantum physics genius that inspired Albert Einstein, is said to have stated, "If you only knew the magnificence of the 3, 6 and 9, then you would hold a key to the universe". The numbers 3, 6, and 9 are the fundamental root vibrations of the Solfeggio frequencies.

These healing frequencies are an expression of the frequencies our energy field vibrates with when we are whole.

The Solfeggio Frequencies are:

174 Hz - Alleviating Stresses
285 Hz - Rejuvenation
396 Hz - Liberating guilt & fear
417 Hz - Healing the past
528 Hz - Miracles
639 Hz - Relationships, Connection & love
741 Hz - Mental Clarity & Solutions
852 Hz - Peace to overthinking
963 Hz - Pineal Gland & Connection to Source

15) Guild remedies - Colours

These can be colour remedies made by Ambika Wauters, or those proved by the Guild. The following are the colour remedies as proved by the Guild.

a) Green

- Shock to the heart centre
- Individual may have shut down completely
- Shock from a past life
- Inertia; fear to incarnate, grow
- Useful with alcoholics along with polycrests
- Huge sadness in the heart
- Lack of love, having been hurt
- Brings compassion towards those who hurt us
- Those who need mothering, nurturing
- Damaged by the father, deserted by the father
- Lots of grief, including for partner
- Can feel hollow
- Calming, restores connection & trust
- Those who abuse or misuse their power
- Nervous anticipation
- Better for the sun, need a lot of sunlight

This is another wonderful remedy for the heart, really connects us with the heart, where there's been shock into the heart centre. It's such a healing remedy that's about opening up to the possibilities. Someone may have shut their heart down completely because of shock or because of trauma, whether it's in this life or another life. There might be an inertia. It's challenging to grow and evolve and move forward. It can be really useful as a remedy for addictions, along with polycrests.

b) Orange

- Purification, stillness & calm
- In the eye of the storm, the point of stillness
- Hugely protective
- Death, birth & transition
- Getting on the right path
- An enable
- Brings movement & the energy for movement forward
- Reconnects us with our path
- Useful when feeling stuck
- Grounding
- Expansiveness into life
- Strengthens the aura
- Closely linked with spiral

I love orange as a remedy. I studied Aura Soma, which is a colour healing system. Vicky Wall, the creator and founder of Aura Soma was a pharmacist who in her later years lost her physical vision, and then started to intuitively see and experience colours. She was a remarkable soul. Vicky Wall taught that orange is a remarkable colour vibration that heals shock and trauma, and it also heals addiction.

I have come to the realisation that the sacral chakra is more important to bring healing to than the root chakra. When people experience shock and trauma, or abuse, we've historically been taught that it's the root chakra that's most affected. People become ungrounded, and they don't feel safe. One of the things that I teach is that actually, when someone needs grounding, it's usually because they don't feel safe. And usually, they don't feel safe because of the impact of somebody else's behaviour.

Each chakra *connects* us with an aspect of life.

The root chakra connects us with physical life, stability and security.

The sacral chakra connects us with relationships with others.

The solar plexus chakra connects us with ourselves; our gifts and our power. And so this is where we can feel our fears; our self-doubts.

A trauma that directly affects the root chakra would be something like an environmental disaster; where people are no longer safe in their physical lives on the Earth.

Abuse however causes trauma to the body, mind and soul through the sacral chakra, because it can only occur through the actions of another human, or a group of humans - in other words, in relationship with others (even if those people are not known to us, we are in relationship with them in some way if their actions have an effect on us). Abuse affects the natural balance of the sacral chakra, and so we can lose trust in other people, and our sense of safety when we are with them. The effect of this ripples down to the root chakra (so we don't feel safe physically and become ungrounded), and ripples up to the solar plexus chakra (so we don't trust ourselves or love ourselves or connect to our power), but it is through damage to the sacral chakra - because of the actions of another - that these effects are felt.

People can turn to addictions in order to fulfil their need to feel loved - where a person couldn't give this to them, then a substance or food might. The sacral chakra is the chakra associated with addictions.

Of course, the effects of abuse can and does travel through all of the chakras, but I wanted to highlight how healing abuse primarily is best done by working through the sacral chakra first.

The sacral chakra has traditionally been seen as being orange in colour. Vicky Wall taught that orange helps us to reintegrate our body, mind and soul when we go into shock.

Orange is a colour that brings healing to shock and trauma, and is one I have found helpful with addictions.

I have found this remedy to be a very motivating remedy to help someone connect with their mojo - and to get onto the right path. Where Golden Spiral brings a beautiful gentle unfolding, Orange - like Milky Way - just like moves someone into place. And this is why I work with Orange plus Milky Way together, usually at high potency, and find it really brings a wonderful shift. Usually I give a 10M if someone's vital force can take it. It's useful when someone feels stuck, helps bring grounding, makes someone very present, so they can start taking a can-do approach in their life.

c) Purple

- Any state of transformation or transition
- Deep depression & anxiety – gives a universal view
- Brings stillness, inner peace & calm
- Power, miracles, magic
- Pregnancy & birth – babies in wrong position, who do not want to incarnate
- Death – both for the person dying & their families
- Blood – all conditions affecting the blood, including anaemia and blood cancers
- Useful for concentration eg on a long drive
- Useful with those with addictions & obsessions
- Useful for healers before facilitating healing sessions

Purple is an incredible remedy for times of transformation or transition. It can bring a healing of deep, deep depression and anxiety. I really got to see it do its work when I was without my son for a year. There were times I just spent days in bed. I just couldn't function sometimes. There being this one time when I'd been in bed for about three days, other than of course, go to the toilet, or get a drink, and I lost a lot of weight. And I remember thinking, about three days in, "hang on a minute, I don't have to stay in this state of like real pain. I've got remedies". I literally crawled to the top of the stairs and slid down the stairs on my belly. I really did feel that bad.

I hadn't worked with Purple many times, but my intuition told me to take a Purple. So I took a 10M. 10 minutes later, I was completely back in my body, fully present, able to stand up and was ready to start taking on living as normally as I could. I felt "normal". I got get in the shower and did normal day-to-day activities. It was so transformative for me. It was like a beautiful wind had been blown through me to just clear away the cobwebs so I could be myself again, as much as it's possible to be yourself in the circumstances I was in at the time.

It's one of the big transition remedies. And as I mentioned earlier, for me, the ones I work with, the Golden Spiral and Purple, it's got magic in it. This remedy has got magic in it, power, miracles and magic.

d) Yellow

- Trauma, especially from abusive father
- Person may not have a strong identity due to father's actions – this remedy helps reconnect that
- Protective in relation to the father
- Brings peace, stillness & reconnects with power
- Useful where there is dependency
- Purification (especially with Clay & Thymus Gland)
- Radiation
- Where Earth has been polluted / damaged by radiation
- Suppression – may appear to be gentle
- Don't believe in own abilities, or trust life
- Expansive remedy
- Female remedy
- Cancer
- Indecisive
- Might be lethargic, have low energy

I find this to be a beautiful remedy to work with in relation to abuse from the father. Colin Griffith also recommends a beautiful combination of Yellow, Clay and Thymus Gland for purification, which I find to be a beautiful mix.

Yellow is the colour of the solar plexus chakra which is the chakra that connects us with our gifts and personal power. When we're in our personal power, we can make decisions effectively. It helps to bring healing there.

16) Guild Remedies - General

a) Ayahuasca

- Brings light where there has been darkness
- Split states; out of the body
- Releasing souls from painful soul contracts
- Life & death remedy
- Children born with the umbilicus around the neck
- A lot of fear; dear of disease, fear of cancer
- Deep grief, deep pain; grief from the beginning of time
- Self-hatred
- Loss of faith & hope
- Loss of memory

I absolutely love this remedy; I just think it's incredible. It is said that the first time you take Ayahuasca in material form can, for some people, be an initiation into facing what it is you need to face in order to become a warrior. And that very much was my experience on the one occasion I took it as part of a shamanic journey, so I have chosen not to do so again.

As a remedy however, I find it to be remarkable. I have repeatedly seen in patients how it welcomes in light. I use it a lot in combinations with other remedies. It combines beautifully with Syphilinum. I used a lovely combination inspired by Nick Biggins of Petrified Sequoia, Ayahuasca and Syphilinum, which is about clearing ancestral trauma, going back to the very beginning of time.

Ayahuasca, I find, is also deeply, deeply clearing. It's another remedy that when people get stuck and they can't see a way forward, Ayahuasca brings the light. There are other remedies that I give to support the momentum and the energy of forward movement such as Golden Spiral, Orange and Milky Way. Ayahuasca, however, shines the way forward.

b) Buddleia

- Clears shock & trauma from the psyche
- Works through lifetimes
- Helps clear karma & ancestral trauma
- Useful where there is still shock from another lifetimes reverberating in this one
- Homeopathic tranquiliser
- Great fear, panic & terror
- Afraid of the dark
- Fear of being oneself
- To support transition in & out of incarnation
- Where someone has detached emotionally
- For children – especially where there has been sexual abuse
- Fathers – lack of father energy in the person's life
- Mental blockages; poor or non development of mental & emotional faculties

- People who want to cry but can't
- Brings light out of the gloom
- Mid life crisis

This is the meditative proving equivalent of aconite in terms of working with shock and trauma. It works through lifetimes and is a big energy remedy, clearing trauma in all its forms. It's another light bringing remedy. It does so in a much gentler way than ayahuasca.

I often use this in combination. Sometimes I give it in combination with aconite, but I often use it in combinations where I'm giving much deeper remedies as a combination when supporting people going through huge traumas.

I'm very blessed to know an incredible family court judge who is fair and understands the importance of dealing with the abusive situations that show up, and so I am lucky to know that there are some good people working in toxic systems. I have met really destructive Judges. There are also really loving, kind, considered Judges. The systems themselves, however, are toxic and patriarchal. They are designed to divide (families) and conquer. I have one patient who was walking through a very intense time in the family court system, and was at risk of losing her child, despite being incredibly loving. Having had my own experiences of just how traumatic and stressful these experiences can be - and intense in ways that are unimaginable - I made a combination of eleven different remedies, all as a 10M mix, just to support, with directions of take one as needed, because there comes a point when I feel that when someone is walking through so much intensity, it's just OK to throw "everything and the kitchen sink" at a prescription just to help the patient get through it. In these situations, people are literally staring at the underbelly of the beast. That was definitely the case for her.

(The combination I gave is: Aconite, Buddleia, Green, Rainbow, Purple, Ayahuasca, Ignatia, Staphysagria, Causticum, Lotus, Rose Quartz Essence.

I also gave a Life Path / Karma Clear mix I have combined at 50M weekly made of: Aquamarine, Berlin Wall, Plutonium, Kigelia, Silver Birch, Petrified Sequoia, Milky Way, Golden Spiral, Flower of Life, Rose, Spectrolite. I didn't have Dodona or Tree of Life then, but I would add both to this now. And I hadn't worked with Chalice Well Water then, but I would consider it now. I also separately prescribed Syphilinum.

She did really well. She felt really supported by the remedies, and several remarkable shifts happened, which she attributed to the remedies. The father massively shifted and they came to an agreement right at the last minute, and he dropped his attempt to have her child taken from her).

c) Butterfly

- Release of darkness, darkest of karmas
- Enormous transformation
- Transitions, growth & development
- Dying & rebirthing
- Heart-opening remedy; removes fear
- Heavy heart, broken after grief & bereavement
- Sadness, depressed, can't see a way forward;stuck
- Those living in the material world cut off from their spirituality
- Mental illness; schizophrenia; separation from Source
- Teenagers where there is confusion & a loss of sense of reality
- For creative people; musicians, poets, artists, who can end up becoming mad
- Can see the greatest potential we can have; connects us to our soul's purpose
- Relationships between the sexes
- Balances masculine & feminine energies
- Wonderful remedy for children incarnating in
- Nervous system remedy (vagus nerve, paralysis, numbness, tingling

Butterfly is such a lovely remedy for helping somebody to be able to move into the next phase of their life and just do it with such a celebration of their own beauty. There are remedies for moving people forward in their life that give them the impetus to move and to shift and transform in their lives. But this is a remedy that does it while celebrating who the person is. There's this real release of moving from having been this heavy caterpillar, crawling along the ground on your belly, and the heaviness of that, to being light and free. So it's a lovely remedy that brings lots of freedom.

d) Chalice Well Water

- Stillness & surrender; the point between heaven & earth, darkness & light
- Takes a person to place of complete surrender
- Corresponds to the winter solstice; when sun dies before it is reborn
- Transitions whether labour or death
- New beginnings
- Much fear
- Extreme lack of self-confidence, fear of criticism – especially from so-called authority
- People afraid of spiritual development, useful for teenagers
- Overwhelmed by emotions – grief
- Spine – enhances flow of CSF
- Fluid – too much fluid in body, flooding of menstrual periods
- Lots of hunger; unfulfilled longing

Chalice well water is quite interesting to me. I've only really started working with it a lot more recently. Glastonbury and Chalice Well in particular is one of my most favourite places in the whole world. The waters are said to have sprung up when some say the brother, others the cousin, of Christ - Joseph of Arimathea - had travelled there and placed his staff in the ground, and a spring of holy sacred waters emerged. So the waters carry the vibration of Christ Consciousness, and also the vibration of Mary Magdalena.

They were members of a tribe called the Essene tribe. The Essenes practiced a form of Judaism, but had been rejected by the mainstream Jewish community, because they were seen as a bit of a cult for two reasons. Firstly, the Essenes practiced equality between the sexes. So men and women were truly equals. Secondly, they didn't use a priest or somebody in a position of power to guide them spiritually, as happens in modern religions. They lived a very deeply spiritual practice, incredibly humbly. They practiced the art of being their own antennae to God, as it were, So what that did was that it meant that they didn't give their power away to an external spiritual leader.

They studied in the temples of Isis in ancient Egypt. They understood the importance of sacred relationships. They taught sacred sexuality. They practiced and lived that. Jesus and Mary Magdalena embodied that in their relationship, which is why they're both such a wonderful beacon of light in terms of sacred relationships. It is said according to some channels that they learned how to reach such elevated vibrations and alignment with Source that some were able to conceive using light. Jesus wasn't the only one of the Essene tribe to have been conceived by light. His mother, Mother Mary, was also said to have been conceived by light also, as were others. So when Joseph of Arimathea went to Glastonbury and is said to put his staff in the ground, he was bringing with him that vibration that the Essenes carried, which was of a true, deep connection with the pure, unconditional love of Source and the sacredness of the expression of life.

Chalice Well is a place of great stillness and peacefulness. The water itself has two different streams. The Well comes through what's known as the red water which is iron rich, and you see it in all of the areas through which the water flows because it's got that kind of reddish brown tinge to it. That's the male water. The female water is called the white water, and doesn't have the same levels of iron, but it's got quite high levels of calcium, so they have to filter out some of that for safety reasons, because excessively high levels of calcium can affect the heart.

I've found this to be an exceptional grief remedy. My main go-to for grief has been Colin Griffith's wonderful combination of Ignatia, Lotus and Rose Quartz. Where Ignatia doesn't go as deeply as is really needed for deep soul levels of grief, I now look to either Cygnus Cygnus, Sandalwood or Chalice Well Water.

It's a very deeply, beautiful, peace bringing remedy.

e) Frankincense

- Gift to baby Jesus & carries the energy of Christ consciousness
- Awakens consciousness
- Reconnects with heart & heart-based wisdom
- Have nearly drowned in this or drowned in a past life
- Light out of the darkness
- Point of completion
- Goes to the dark night of the soul & brings the person out to the light
- For those who can't take any more, feel suicidal
- Great trauma & tragedy
- Purifies, energises, relaxes
- For stress that people don't know how to deal with
- Low, irritable, depressed
- Brings great peace
- Fun & laughter
- Lots of abundance in the stillness
- Remedy for death & dying

Frankincense was, of course, a gift to the baby Jesus and so carries the vibration of Christ consciousness. Most people use sage when they want to clear their homes energetically. I find frankincense to be much more powerful than sage in house clearing. I burn the resin on heated charcoal discs.

f) Lotus

- Carries Buddha energy & the energy of angels
- Universal healer
- For sceptics, wakes people up
- Brings forgiveness for self & others
- Surrendering to the will of the Divine ("Thy will be done")
- Cancer
- Facilitates movement
- New beginnings
- Death & dying
- Forgetfulness
- Ego-centric, focused on looking good; vanity
- Low self-esteem, feeling ugly
- Feel like a failure, may go on to develop cancer
- Traumatic birth, despair at having a disabled child
- Locked into grief

I love this remedy. It is in the Colin Griffith grief triad of Ignatia, Lotus and Rose quartz. It's like adding a hug in a bottle. It's another what I call an "outbreath" remedy; it invites the exhale; a release of something, a letting go; a relaxation.

g) Milky Way

- Link with the Divine
- Great expansion
- Removes blocks to connecting with Divine love and laughter
- Connection with the Universe
- Unifying, heals relationships
- Carries light around the body
- Connection & communication
- For those not on their path
- Can be high achievers or under achievers
- Have great power but may not be using it; may be afraid of it
- Need lots of support
- Nervous system support
- Impatience
- Sense of loss
- Can find it hard to receive love yet demand it

I love working with Milky Way. The Milky Way is an expression of the Golden Spiral just in the galaxy and/or the galaxies that flow through the Milky Way. So it really helps to move people forward and through and align them in the natural unfolding journey of their life.

I use this when someone has got stuck in their lives. I can give Golden Spiral which moves through gently. If someone needs a bit of a rocket fuel blast moving forward, then what I will also give is Milky Way along with Orange. really like those two remedies together.

h) Rainbow

- Hugely purifying
- Suicidal depression
- Connects the corpus callosum – the bridge between the two halves of the brain
- Where psyche is divided (eg schizophrenia)
- People feeling disconnected
- People who have experienced abuse
- People who never feel safe, who keep moving on rather than put down roots
- Combats radiation
- Useful for teenagers

Rainbow is hugely purifying. It's in one of the remedies in a beautiful combination that the Guild put together for clearing chemo and radiation that is available at Helios. It's such a beautiful remedy for doing cleansing and detoxing.

When somebody needs to make a shift to feel like there's something positive and beautiful in their life and that they can just reach into and over and cross that seemingly impossible-to-cross bridge, Rainbow is a wonderful remedy. It creates that bridge over from one state or one place to the next.

i) Silver Birch

- This is a tree or magic & protection; it heals & harmonises
- Release of karma
- Karmic states where people have been pushed to the limit, broken down, are full of fear & weariness
- Expansive vibration – draws people out of those karmic states
- Brings change & movement, release
- Release of pain & burdens
- For years of hurt & grief, years of crying
- Brings peace & tranquility
- Purification – including of kidneys & skin
- Releases female energies where these have been suppressed
- Complete exhaustion, wiped out
- Cannot concentrate
- Stuck – unblocks
- Support for autoimmune illnesses, boosts immune system

I love this remedy. I give this remedy quite a lot when I'm working with people who have got lots of ancestral karma or personal karma. I tend to give a triad of Petrified Sequoia (New Earth, not Meditative Proving Sequoia), Syphilinum and Ayahuasca on one day in the week, often Monday, and Silver Birch on another day, often Thursday, in higher potencies (10M if the patient can handle it)

It's another "outbreath" remedy - it helps people let go. It's another light bringing remedy. It brings lightness to a person in their life. As a tree, the Silver Birch has magic in it and protection. This remedy clears karma and then enables somebody to expand and pulls people out of those karmic states into where they are in the here and the now. It brings positive change and movement - I see that when I work with it. It brings this sense of release.

j) Stonehenge

- Connects with the soul and with Source
- Welcomes in light
- Aligns the chakras
- A transition remedy
- For those that do not wish to be here
- Reconnects with purpose, vision, the will, courage and the energy to move forwards
- For those who have experienced considerable pain
- Welcomes peace and tranquility

17) Guild Remedies - Crystals

There are also crystal remedies made by, and proved by Peter Tuminello.

The following are ones I use that have been proved by the Guild.

a) Aquamarine

- Soothes the heart & soul
- Like Arnica for the soul
- Deep family (ancestral) trauma & grief
- Peace where there has been conflict within
- Shock & trauma to the psyche
- Sadness & grief
- Haunted by the past
- Heaviness of years of emotional turmoil
- May need solitude
- Desolation, hopelessness, staring into the void
- Suicidal thoughts
- Damaged aura
- Find it hard to stay in the present
- Feeling one cannot cope with any more traumas
- Can support the work of other heart remedies

This is one remedy to consider when someone is so stuck and you just don't know where to go with them - and perhaps other remedies aren't yet working, yet they may be exhausted by the traumas in their life. And they feel so like just everything feels too much and they need to find a way out and a way forward.

It's interesting to me that it has suicidal thoughts in its picture. I don't give this as a first thought remedy where someone is feeling suicidal. We know Aurum as a first consideration when someone is feeling suicidal, but I'm always interested in the reason why someone is feeling suicidal and what has taken them to that point.

I once had a really fantastic conversation with a psychotherapist where we were talking about how in the traditional medical model approach to suicidal feelings, it's pathologised. Feeling suicidal is seen as a dis-ease and illness in some way, shape or form, and is treated as a mental illness. The psychotherapist I spoke to explained that everybody at some point has the capacity to feel suicidal, if they've lost enough that matters to them in their life. For some people, it might not take a lot, they might only lose what to some of us may seem like a relatively small amount, and for others, they may lose everything and still not feel suicidal and keep walking forward. Everyone however has something that will push them to that point where they just think they can't carry on.

As well as being interested in what has pushed someone to that point, 'm also interested in whether there are any ancestral stories; any links to any family history around death – or mass deaths – in terms of war trauma, perhaps. Then I look to the big ancestral remedies. In working with Family Constellations, I have seen how sometimes it can be that someone is carrying the grief of ancestors who lost many loved ones in war, and the surviving ancestor carried survivor's guilt which is a trauma that is passed down and can cause a descendant to carry the feeling of wishing to be dead. In the cases, it's often unexplainable. This is when working with one or more of the big ancestral trauma remedies could be really helpful.

b) Amethyst

- Deeply cleansing of the heart chakra
- Grief that goes back a long way
- Encourages the patient to tell the truth
- Addictions
- Protection & purification
- Clears the energy field
- Insomnia
- Out of body states – brings us back

I find this to be such a beautiful remedy. It's deeply, deeply cleansing. Amethyst is a crystal that's hugely protective and is cleansing.

There might be addictions, there might be a need for protection and purification, which is usually my main reason for choosing amethyst.

It is a remedy to consider for insomnia. If our energy fields are too open, then we may go into lucid dreaming, or into out of body states. We might be astral traveling. We might be really busy when we're sleeping, which can make it very difficult to get restful sleep. Amethyst is a remedy that helps clear our energy field so that when we are going to bed, we're not dealing with all sorts of energies everywhere in the same way, as well as bringing us back to our bodies.

It's a remedy that brings us back to our bodies differently to how the tree remedies work. The tree remedies are very solidifying, very grounding. Amethyst just calls us back to be whole. I really like this remedy for cleansing.

c) Ametrine

- A combination of amethyst & citrine
- Those who find changes hard due to grief stuck at the Thymus centre
- Nervous system repair, including the brain
- Memory loss & trauma following war & violence – CPTSD
- Feeling crushed
- Hidden trauma & abuse
- Pain from sexual abuse
- Huge pain held in throat & thymus
- Tremendous grief
- MS, cerebral palsy, MND, stroke, accident
- Not being able to make the body do what you want it to do
- Sense of isolation

- Feeling unworthy
- Self-harm & cutting

I have found to be a fantastic remedy. I haven't used it many times, but when I have, it's been so deeply clearing. It's a big trauma remedy in all sorts of ways, maybe where there's hidden trauma, maybe where there's been abuse, maybe there's been sexual abuse and people are finding it difficult to move on. It brings in the wonderful cleansing aspects of amethyst, the purification of the energy field and the protection of the energy field, with the deep cleansing of citrine, which also welcomes greater abundance and joy.

It's a remedy that revives. It reconnects people back to themselves so that they can start to move forward again. What I've seen it do for patients is it's almost like everything comes back online again, their brain, their brain function, their energy field, and they feel clearer and more present.

Self-harm and cutting come from a need to release intense emotions that somebody is struggling with. What I experience when someone gets to that point is that their energy field is no longer clear. It may be that they have what are known as earthbound spirits or attachments, depending on what your school of thinking is. It basically means that in the same way that on Earth, there are people who are lovely and really kind and other people who are traumatised, and have gone into a difficult place in terms of their behaviour or their thinking, or are unhappy. Maybe people develop addictions because they're struggling to cope. When we pass into spirit, we have the same mirror. Just like in the film Ghost, apart from the spirits that come for Carl, that is an excellent depiction of what can happen. The illustration of how Sam, Patrick Swayze's character, is killed suddenly, the light appears for him to go back to Source, but he doesn't want to leave his body or his girlfriend Molly. So the light appears, he doesn't go into it, and then he ends up stuck here. He finds he's got work to do, and they expose Carl before the light appears again at the end of the film, because he is ready to go back to Source.

As people transition into spirit, if they don't take the opportunity to step into connecting with the incredible light that appears - the pure unconditional love of Source - then they can become what's called earthbound.

Some energy healers help those earthbound spirits go back to Source. It's quite common that when someone passes, they don't want to leave their children. So they stay without understanding that if they go to the light, they can have their healing with Source and then come back again. They worry that they might have to leave their children and never be able to return. If they go to the pure unconditional love of Source and have a healing from all that they've carried in their life, they can come back out of choice to be with their families, and they do so from a truly healed space. So they can actually help so much more, but so many people don't know that.

Many earthbound spirits still carry their traumas in their personality cloak and the tiredness from their own life, whilst they're still trying to help their families on earth, because they don't go back to Source. In the same way that we have people who can behave in really problematic ways on earth, when they pass into spirit, they can still remain like that. If someone has an addiction when they pass, they can go to seek somebody who also has a similar addiction and just hang around that person so that they can get a bit of the energy hit whenever the addict is using whatever substance they are addicted to.

So there are all sorts of different ways in which people's energy fields can become unclear, or they can have attachments or earthbound spirits.

I'm very fortunate in that I come from a a healing background where we take a positive view in that this is an opportunity to support those spirits being able to return back to Source. It's really important to have training with somebody who's really trustworthy, that really is aligned with the pure, unconditional love of Source in every way in which they work. There are plenty of healers who can teach that kind of work, but they don't do it through the pure, unconditional love of Source first, which is the safest way to do this work. And that is the ultimate protection, that's the ultimate healing.

I also think it's really important in saying all of this to share that I don't judge people for having attachments. I've seen a lot of judgment in spiritual circles for it, and lots of, "Oh, that person isn't clear, their energy field isn't clear." We don't go around on purpose trying to collect difficult energies. So for me, there's no judgment around it. I have found it useful with friends I know, love and trust who do this work too, every now and then to just check each other's energy fields to see if they need to be cleared. We can't always see it or sense it for ourselves - in fact, it can be very difficult sometimes to sense for ourselves.

The reason I say all of this is that Ametrine is one of the remedies that is good at clearing the energy field. I would suggest that self-harm and cutting is an expression of having an unclear energy field.

I would suggest there is something that needs healing and releasing from the energy field; someone who is self-harming and cutting has gone into quite a dark place. It may be an Earthbound spirit. The spirit might be an ancestors and that is often the work of Family Constellations - to bring peace to ancestors who are still troubled due to traumas in their lives that were never healed.

Ametrine is helpful at clearing and protecting the energy field through the amethyst whilst bringing the vibration of joy and lightness through the citrine. ,

d) Emerald

- Too much or not enough ego
- Can be haughty, arrogant or overly humble & have a great lack of confidence
- Nervous system; all aspects
- Cancer
- Trauma especially where knocked out of body by trauma
- Radiation
- Throat
- Blocked or low energy
- Reawakens spark of life where spirit is becoming sad & tired of life
- Shattered dreams
- Wakes with vengeful thoughts
- Poorly nourished, not assimilating
- Allergies
- Cleansing of drugs eg HRT, anaesthetic

I often use this in combination when detoxing allopathic drugs, especially where chemotherapy or radiation are involved. I also find it a really lovely remedy for helping patients draw boundaries in unhealthy relationships - it's like a more present version of Carcinosin to me in that way.

e) Obsidian

- Cleansing from drugs (pharmaceutical, recreational, pollution, smoking, alcohol, toxicity in general)
- Energy clearing
- Dispels negative forces & protects the aura
- Protection & grounding for children & babies
- Despair & depression
- May look on the dark side; like wading through treacle
- Fear of moving forwards, anxiety
- Calm on the outside, but turmoil on the inside
- Calming for the adrenals
- Want to be part of life, but feel blocked in some way
- Start things but don't finish them
- Suppressed emotions especially anger

Obsidian is a crystal that is used to cleanse and protect the aura. The same is true of it as a remedy. I find this to be a really helpful remedy for energy protection and clearing the energy field, and also for clearing the impact of drugs including pharmaceutical drugs, or recreational drugs.

One patient I had worked as a musician in pubs and bars, but found it difficult to cope with the behaviours of some of the people when drunk. I gave obsidian to take before going to work. She found that it had such a powerful effect - that whenever she took it, she felt completely safe.

f) Rose Quartz

- Reluctance & grief at having incarnated; in being here
- Manic depressive states
- Inability to forgive, hardness
- Can be cruel to others / animals
- Isolated, unappreciated
- Lac of connection, fear of people, desire to be alone
- Daydreams; difficult concentrating, being focused
- Lots of anxiety
- Hidden anger
- Cannot finish things
- Can be panicky
- MS & ME
- Purifies immune system, nervous system, kidneys, lungs, liver, blood, thymus
- Cleanses from radiation, pharmaceutical drugs
- Eczema

Rose Quartz is a crystal that is about healing and opening the heart, and as a remedy, Rose Quartz does the same.

There can be a feeling isolated, feeling unappreciated; a sense of being separate. We had Goldfish and we had Berlin Wall - these remedies are about that sense of being separate from others. This is another remedy to consider in those situations.

I particularly like this remedy for it's cleansing properties, and have seen it work beautifully in some cases of eczema. I only give it alongside other remedies, to support the cleansing process.

18) The 8 Core Chakra Remedies

We have been taught that there are 7 core chakras, however, by adding in an 8th, at the Higher Heart (or Thymus Gland), we connect with an octave according to Pythagorean principles. An octave generates harmonia according to Pythagoras. Also, adding in this additional chakra brings with it a mathematical ratio, Phi (1.618) – found in the Golden Spiral, which is an expression of the flow of all aligned energy and life. This isn't present when working with only 7 chakras.[29]

I would suggest that these are also sarcode remedies.

Root Chakra
Sacral Chakra
Solar Plexus Chakra
Heart Chakra
Thymus Chakra
Throat Chakra
Third Eye Chakra
Crown Chakra

19) Pure Consciousness

This is pure Source / Consciousness / Goddess / God. energy; pure unconditional love. For the trauma of separation from Source.

---

[29] Danica Apolline-Matić (2024) Nature's Medicine Code Second Edition - Danica Apolline-Matić

Prescribing according to the Blueprint Method

The Blueprint Method can be used in one of two ways:

1) As a stand-alone way of prescribing.

For example, just giving one or more of the remedies described here.

The prescription may be as simple as Golden Spiral 30c daily, or may be a combination of remedies, prescribed using any other methods of prescribing.

2) In addition to any other method of prescribing.

For example, using the Triad Method, and then adding Golden Spiral 30c daily.

Case Studies

Case Study 1 - MW

French woman in her 40s. Mother. Several autoimmune conditions - lupus, myosotis, Hashimotos, Raynauds. Extreme fatigue. Digestive issues. Taking methoxetrate, mepacrine, prednisolone, rituximab IVs, antidepressants, has been on steroids for 20 years. Fully COVID vaccinated. Regular infections and antibiotics.

Married husband from different background, hid relationship with him for several years before telling family.

Also history of anorexia. Although in early consults this wasn't mentioned more than once - patient's focus was on the fatigue and autoimmunity so treatment focus went there.

No response to bowel nosodes, lanthanides, working with sarcodes (bone marrow, blood cells, spleen, liver, mitochondria), detox protocols, grief remedies, Nat Mur, Ignatia, Arsenicum, Nux, Carc, Syph, Thuja.

Then in one session, just as she was about to give up, she mentioned the anorexia in passing for only the second time.

Re-repping led me to Tarentula hisp. I asked her if she loved music and dancing and whether she just had to dance when music came on. She started to cry about how much she missed dancing, how it's her favourite thing in the world. I thought about her hiding her relationship.

I prescribed Tarentula hisp 200c twice daily with Phos Ac.

Following session she describes having had a breakdown. Daily trips to A&E, begging for tests. Thought she had cancer and was dying. Suicidal. Was writing goodbye letters.

I prescribed Aurum 10M daily for three days then weekly plus Golden Spiral 1M daily.

Following session, for the first time in years:

Felt better, her energy was better, muscles started working better, she had been EATING, had gained weight, had a trial session with a therapist that went well, talked to doctor about coming off antidepressants who supported her wish, found her mojo, felt like a different person, and decided she was refusing to be ill anymore.

Further treatments and tests continued, and she decided not to continue with homeopathy, however her vital force had become activated.

Case Study 2 - KS

This patient and her 11 year old daughter were living with her parents. The relationship with her parents has been abusive and toxic for her whole life. Furthermore, they don't understand her spirituality. She felt that she didn't really have a family she could look to or rely upon. She had had several relationships that were abusive / toxic. She is a highly sensitive person. She was struggling to cope with the family situation. KS wanted greater freedom from them, and a clearer direction in her life. She felt trapped and tied to her family whilst being desperate to leave.

I prescribed:

Petrified Sequoia / Ayahuasca 10M Mondays
Carc 1M Thursdays
Golden Spiral 30c daily

KS took the Petrified Sequoia / Ayahuasca and Golden Spiral on a Monday when the remedies arrived. On the Tuesday, she was contacted by a long lost cousin she hadn't seen in 35 years. They met that Friday with her long lost aunt and uncle, and KS felt that she had been reconnected with the family that she had always dreamed of.

Over the following 10 months, we worked with:

Petrified Sequoia / Ayahuasca
Anacardium
Carcinosin
Thuja
Golden Spiral
Goldfish
Matridonal remedies
Columba
Butterfly
Flower of Life, Stramonium & Rose

By the end of the 10 months, she had found her way to balance, with clearer energy, clearer thinking, greater groundedness and self-reliance. She got to the stage where she felt able to leave her family situation and move to Portugal, which she had dreamed of doing with her daughter. She is now living a happy life there.

Case Studies 3

3 cases of the recent difficult to treat cases of the outbreak of coughs / whooping cough. Pertussin 1M gave some relief, as did Drosera 200c as needed in each case. One responded to Phosphorus 1M, but the effect did not last.

Other remedies had been tried to no avail, including Ant-tart and Kennel Cough Nosode.

In each of these 3 cases, I gave Flower of Life plus Golden Spiral 50M and immediately in each case, breathing became easier, the person became calmer, a reduction in frequency and duration of coughing happened straight away, and the symptoms continued to ease over the following 3-5 days.

Case Studies 4 - Detoxification 1

I use tautopathy / human chemistry with a great love for it, especially when detoxing hormones, steroids, metals, fungi, moulds and antibiotics.

Using the COVID vaccines in potency was the first point in time for me where I strongly felt that the vibration of the remedies was just too low for me to give to patients. I did try with one patient, but it just intuitively felt "dirty" to me.

It was at this point that I started working with a combination of Golden Spiral, Thuja & Silica 30c three times a day for 5-7 days and daily for another 21 days later. I have since added Flower of Life, since making and proving the remedy, so I give a combination of:

Golden Spiral
Flower of Life
Thuja
Silica

30c three times a day for 5-7 days and daily for another 21 days.

I have consistently seen an improvement in the health of each patient that has ever been given this protocol. I have been contacted by two kinesiologists, independently, who didn't know each other, and one homeopath who also tested this, and all said they were testing that this protocol works.

I have repeatedly seen patients love taking it so much, that they feel more peace with themselves, and in their lives, they ask if they can continue taking it after they have finished the protocol.

In two cases, patients made significant life changes, choosing a new career in each case whilst taking this combination. I always tell patients working with this protocol that they can continue taking the remedies as long as they feel they would like to, and that if their intuition tells them they have taken enough and to stop, to listen to that.

I find patients do not prove or aggravate this combination.

Case Studies 5 - Detoxification 2

When using Ton Jansen's Human Chemistry approach, I now give either:

a) Golden Spiral, Flower of Life, Thuja & Silica 30c as the Saturday remedy, or
b) Flower of Life and Golden Spiral 50M as the Saturday remedy

I consistently find this combination really moves patients through the detoxification process.

About Danica

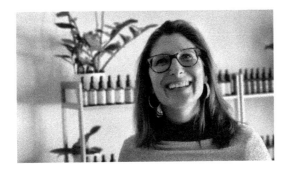

Danica (pronounced De-nit-sa) is a homeopath, writer, blogger, thought leader and health visionary. She is a homeopath, Founder of the Blueprint Essences® and Principal of The Golden Spiral International School of Homeopathy®.

She is also a training specialist, coach, energy healer, baker and entrepreneur. Her passion is health – for the mind, body, soul, within communities and for our beautiful planet.

Danica's other books include The Spiritual Teacher's Handbook, Nature's Medicine Code, Born Feisty and Trauma: a new approach.

She lives in Lewes, England with her son.

www.danicaapollinematic.com
www.goldenspiralschoolofhomeopathy.com
www.blueprintessences.com